DOCUMENTA OPHTHALMOLOGICA

PROCEEDINGS SERIES

VOL. V

Editor

HAROLD E. HENKES

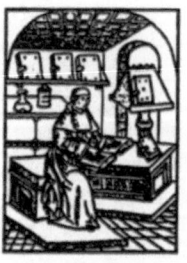

DR. W. JUNK B.V. PUBLISHERS, 1975
THE HAGUE   THE NETHERLANDS

PUBLIC HEALTH OPHTHALMOLOGY

Papers Presented at the Conference on the Prevention
of Impaired Vision and Blindness, Paris, France, May, 1974

Edited by

WILLIAM JOHN HOLMES, M.D.

Secretary General, International Association for
Prevention of Blindness
Honolulu, Hawaii

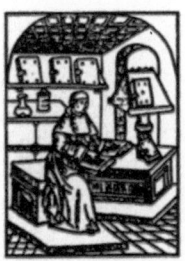

Dr. W. JUNK B.V. PUBLISHERS, 1975
THE HAGUE   THE NETHERLANDS

ISBN-13: 978-90-6193-145-4   e-ISBN-13: 978-94-010-1950-7
DOI: 10.1007/978-94-010-1950-7

IV

CONTENTS

INTRODUCTION

Each year the improvements in communication and transportation, the growing awarness that the resources of this earth are finite, the realization that the population explosion in any part of the world is a concern of all, and the increased economic interdependence of all countries, have increased importance of internationalism as opposed to nationalism. One of the first segments of our society to ignore political and geographic boundaries was that of medicine, particularly in the field of communicable diseases. Valient efforts have been made by some individuals at great personal sacrifice and by individual societies or organizations to prevent and cure blindness and to rehabilitate those who have lost their sight. Only recently, however, have such efforts been consolidated into a major international force. In 1969 the 22nd World Health Assembly of WHO adapted a resolution requesting the Director-General to undertake a study on the information which is at present available on the extent and/or causes of preventable and curable blindness. In 1972 a working group was convened by the World Health Organization in Geneva to outline an attack on the prevention of blindness. At the Paris meeting of the International Congress of Ophthalmology in July of 1974, Mr. JOHN WILSON, who for many years had been one of the leaders in the prevention and cure of blindness on an international basis through his organization of the Royal Commonwealth Society for the Blind, was elected President of the International Association for Prevention of Blindness. He was voted authority to reorganize this association into an effective instrument for attacking the problems of blindness on an international level. He has very rapidly merged the efforts of the World Council for the Blind, the International Association for Prevention of Blindness, and the various national organizations for the prevention of blindness into the International Agency for Prevention of Blindness. Through his amazing organizational ability, strong financial support is developing from many sources. The interest and willingness to support this international effort has been aroused in many professionals, especially the ophthalmologists, and experts in the field of public health medicine.

The symposium on public health ophthalmology held under the sponsorship of the International Association for Prevention of Blindness in Paris in 1974 is an excellent presentation of the importance and immensity of the problems that lie ahead of us in preventing blinding eye disease on an international basis. It gives a new dimension to the speciality of ophthalmology and offers exciting challenges to those interested in the administrative and medical aspects of public health. Dr. WILLIAM JOHN HOLMES is to be thanked and congratulated for his efforts in organizing and editing the material presented at this symposium.

As the efforts of international public health ophthalmology gain momentum many other such symposia will be necessary, for it is only through the publication of such material that the vast number of persons interested in these problems can be informed of the progress that is being made.

A. EDWARD MAUMENEE M.D.

Director
The Wilmer Institute
Johns Hopkins Hospital

PREFACE

At the XXIInd International Congres of Ophthalmology held in Paris, the following resolution, introduced by PROFESSOR G.B. BIETTI, was unanimously approved by both the International Council of Ophthalmology and the International Federation of Ophthalmologic Societies:

As society turns from its past interest, which has been almost exclusively that of curing diseases in individuals, towards concern for preserving and promoting the health of populations, the science of ophthalmology must also increasingly direct its interest towards the public health aspects of eye health.

The field of public health ophthalmology, as a newly emerging concept, offers many opportunities for research and practice of comprehensive eye-health care which includes, in a continuum, prevention, treatment and rehabilitation. It is not, it should not and it cannot be considered as a sub-specialty. It is a new dimension of ophthalmology as a science and a service.

It is considered necessary to develop rapidly this aspect of ophthalmology at the national and international level by:

1. issuing national policy statements for the field of ophthalmology;

2. strengthening the professional dialogue with the disciplines which are relevant to this approach (epidemiology, health administration biostatistics, etc.);

3. promoting the inclusions of public health aspects in ophthalmological curricula; and

4. including public health ophthalmology in the agenda of national, regional and international societies' meetings.

This resolution is timely as there are many ways available for its implementation.

Modern medical and surgical discoveries, improved methods of communication and transportation, emphasis on adequate nutrition and sanitation, the use of the mass media, increasing involvement of allied health peronnel provide means to prevent blindness and impaired vision on an unprecedented global scale.

The successful efforts of Dr. A. EDWARD MAUMENEE of the U.S. and Mr. JOHN WILSON of the U.K. in persuading the World Health Organization to include prevention of blindness within its sphere of activities were a cornerstone of modern public health ophthalmology. The further affiliation of the International Association for the Prevention of Blindness with UNICEF, ILO, the World Council for the Welfare of the Blind and its affiliates, the successful Jerusalem Seminar on the prevention of Blindness held in 1971, and the Paris Conference on the Prevention of Impaired Vision and Blindness held in 1974 were additional building blocks for present-day public health ophthalmology.

Contributors to this volume are principally ophthalmologists from the five continents. Their work was based on clinical experience as well as the untiring efforts of scholars and scientists from a wide array of disciplines that include biochemistry, virology, genetics, nutrition, circulation, and a host of others.

Prevention of blindness from trachoma and diabetic involvement of the eyes is not included in this volume. These subjects were included on the agenda of the XXIInd International Congress of Ophthalmology and will be published in the ACTA of that Congress.

This summary of prevailing concepts, techniques, mass delivery of eye health care, and research in Public Health Ophthalmology around the world is offered with the hope that it will serve as still another cornerstone for the prevention of needless blindness in future generations.

WILLIAM JOHN HOLMES, M.D.

MOBILIZATION OF PUBLIC OPINION IN PUBLIC HEALTH OPHTHALMOLOGY

JOHN WILSON

(Hayward's Heath, Sussex, England)

To mobilize public opinion in public health ophthalmology, may I emphasize three points:

First, there is the need for public awareness of the massive and growing problem of needless blindness and the consequences of any failure to take effective action before population growth makes that problem almost insoluble. Secondly, there are the resources which need to be mobilized if we are to undertake this task in more than a marginal sense. Finally, the implication of all this for the international organizations concerned, the need for expansion, for coordination and for a world view of priorities.

The broad facts are not in dispute. There are at least fifteen million blind people in the world and unless decisive action is taken, there could be thirty million by the end of this century. In the developing countries, where numbers are growing most rapidly, most of this blindness is preventible and much of it is curable.

In human terms the cost of blindness is incalculable. In economic terms it is astonishing, mounting to an annual budget exceeding one billion dollars simply for rehabilitation, welfare and basic maintenance. In the developing countries, rehabilitation extends only to a minute fraction of the blind and those of us who are concerned internationally with blind welfare look with horror at the prospect of new burdens totally beyond foreseeable resources.

This is already happening on a scale exceeding our worst expectation. Two years ago in Bangladesh 100,000 children are estimated to have gone blind from xerophthalmia. In India there may now be four million people blind from cataract. Beyond this there are the awesome statistics of eye disease — twenty million people affected by onchocerciasis, five hundred million by trachoma.

We know these facts but they are not part of that general awareness which forms public opinion and generates political and administrative action. The specialists are concerned, but the case for action has not yet been sufficiently made to people who set national priorities and design development plans — the Prime Ministers, The Ministers, the political and administrative leaders, the legislators. This, I believe, is why even in those countries where there is a compelling case for immediate action, the prevention of blindness fails to receive the priority it so obviously deserves.

It will not be easy to attract attention in a world drenched and numbed with statistics. The prevention of blindness has, for too long, been presented as a medical specialism or a bi-product of welfare concerned with un-

1

pronounceable diseases like onchocerciasis and xerophthalmia. Yet, essentially, it is concerned with immediate human realities − a child blind for lack of green vegetables, a community at risk because there are blinding flies in the river. The time has perhaps come when, adding together the insights of all our disciplines, we can present this need in its broad, understandable human outline − not just as a technique, a subject, but as a cause and a movement generating mass interest, expressing itself through national plans and the co-ordinated programmes of international agencies.

The causes of blindness have been sufficiently identified and there is no doubt that, given the resources and personnel, it would be possible in the next two decades to control the diseases which produce most of the blindness in the developing world. Obviously, there is a need for intensive research, for surveys and the demonstration of new techniques − subjects which at present dominate the agendas of our international conferences. They are, I venture to think, secondary in importance to the mobilization of resources and the need to achieve that coordination of structures and philosophies which can transcend the boundaries of separate disciplines and set our objective within the significant movements and aspirations of our age.

The resources which are required look formidable when measured against the total inadequacy of the resources at present available. They are not if we measure them against the scale of benefits which will result or even against the cost of inaction. What is it worth to a country such as Indonesia to save 10.000 children a year from nutritional blindness − or to India restore sight each year to another half million people blinded by cataract? Just such calculations were made recently by the World Bank in assessing the economic value of controlling onchocerciasis in West Africa; because that program was justified in terms of cost effectiveness, millions of dollars became available.

What would be the cost of coordinated action throughout the developing world to control, over the next 25 years, onchocerciasis, xerophthalmia, trachoma and cataract, and so to break the link between blindness and population growth? In terms of national and international budgets the cost would be large but it would not be astronomical and, given a sufficient movement of international opinion, it would, I am convinced, not be unobtainable. If that cost is not paid now in rational planning and coordinated action, the bill will not go away; at compound interest it will return to be paid in mounting economic loss, in human frustration, in the stunted lives of children.

Only the United Nations and its specialized agencies, acting with member governments, has the capacity to generate and deploy resources on that scale. Already the ground work has been laid in the resolutions of the World Health Assembly, and in the action of WHO, UNICEF and others. Beyond this point even these world giants can act only in response to national requests within a sympathetic climate of opinion.

It is the indispensable role of the non-governmental agencies to create that climate and the conditions within which large scale governmental action becomes possible. To do this, we must be capable of developing our own resources and of concerting them within a movement which is large

2

enough to influence international opinion and to promote national action. It must be broad enough to comprehend every relevant discipline and organization. It must command sufficient funds to demonstrate its policies and to make a significant contribution to the prevention and cure of blindness on a global scale.

During the past three months, the international organizations concerned with blindness and its prevention, have been discussing ways in which such an organization could be established and exploring the support it might receive internationally. Already, there is agreement on objectives and a large measure of accord about the type of organization required.

The World Council for the Welfare of the Blind — with its constituent organizations in over 60 countries, supports this action and will participate in any realistic international effort to prevent and cure blindness. The leadership of the International Council of Ophthalmology has welcomed the initiative and is participating in the discussions. The International Association for the Prevention of Blindness — with its associated organizations and its long history of dedication to this cause — has a unique contribution to make to any such development. It might, indeed, serve as the nucleus of the new enterprise.

BLINDNESS IN INDONESIA

J.H.A. MANDANG

(Manado, North Sulawesi, Indonesia)

INTRODUCTION

Indonesia, being a developing country, is still facing poverty. The annual income per capita is US $ 100.00. Inadequate food supplies, lack of knowledge, education, and medico-hygienical facilities, increasing high birth rate — 30 per thousand — are the well-known problems of developing countries.

POPULATION

According to the 1971 Population Census, the Indonesian population is 119,2 million. Indonesia ranks fifth after China, India, the USSR and the United States of America. The age incidence of the Indonesian population is as follows:

0 – 20 years	63.6 million (53.7%)
20 – 65 years	52.6 million (43.8%)
65 years and older	3 million (2.5%)

The consumptive group — 0-20 years and older — is about 56.2%. In the year 2000 the population is expected to reach 235 million.

NUTRITION

According to the National Sample Survey of 1963-1964, the Indonesian's daily menu is very poor. It includes 0.5 kg rice of inferior quality, one chicken per 1-1/2 years, one egg per 2 months, and one liter of milk per year for each person.

EDUCATION

According to the 1971 Census, 93% of the population above 10 years of age have only primary school education or do not attend school at all.

HYGIENE AND SANITATION

According to the 1971 Census, 18 million (90%) houses do not have toilets that fulfill even minimal sanitary requirements; 14 million (70%) houses are

5

without a floor; 12 million (60%) houses do not have good drinking water; and 2.2 million families are living as guests in the houses of relatives.

Poverty, lack of knowledge, and lack of education are responsible for poor medico-hygienic environment.

ILLNESS – 1973

The morbidity rate is 46 per thousand. The majority of illness occurs in children, especially between 0-4 years of age. The commonest causes of illness are infections of the respiratory apparatus, skin infection, gastroenteritis, malaria, and eye diseases.

The mortality rate is 20 per thousand, mostly affecting children with acure enteritis and infection of respiratory apparatus.

The high birth rate, lack of education and knowledge, infection, and malnutrition are common causes of blindness.

INCIDENCE OF BLINDNESS

Blindness data is available from the latter decades of the 19th century. On the basis of visual acuity, 1/60, the general incidence of blindness is 0.8%. This means that in a population of 125 million, there are one million blind. Most of them live in Java and Madura, accounting for 70% of the total Indonesian population.

CAUSES OF BLINDNESS

In Java and Madura, trachoma, xerophthalmia, gonococcal conjunctivitis, variola bulbi, acute conjunctivitis with corneal complications, iritis and iridocyclitis are the most commonest causes. Glaucoma, senile cataract, and other fundus diseases occur at the same frequency as in other countries. Outside Java and Madura, the role of trachoma and xerophthalmia as blinding diseases is low. Most of the blindness in Java and Madura is caused by trachoma and xerophthalmia. Those blinded by xerophthalmia are mostly preschool children.

The trachoma incidence in Java and Madura is 20-25%. One-fourth of this incidence represents malignant forms of trachoma. Outside Java and Madura, trachoma occurs in about 5-8% of the population. Xerophthalmia incidence in Java and Madura is 20-25%, mostly in pre-school children. Outside Java and Madura, the percentage is 3.5.

Trachoma in school-aged children is seen in about 25-30% with spontaneous healing en mass. One-fourth of all trachoma in Java and Madura is malignant, causing palpebral and corneal deformities, ending in blindness due to dense corneal scars, panophthalmitis, or atrophia bulbi.

Infection and malnutrition are the most important causes of blindness in Java and Madura. They are the aftermath of centuries of poverty, lack of knowledge and education, insufficient medico-hygienic facilities, with high population densities.

6

CAMPAIGN AGAINST BLINDNESS

Eliminating poverty by increasing general welfare and annual income per capita, healthier nutrition, increasing and spreading education, fighting and prevention of the infection by improving general hygiene and public health are the obvious solutions to these problems.

Periodic checkups of school children for trachoma and other eye diseases are highly recommended.

Prevention of xerophthalmia by providing high doses of vitamin A to all pre-school-age children orally or by injection.

Using red palm oil in the villages planted by the village people themselves; instruction to food factories on fortifying certain foods with vitamin A.

Glaucoma surveys in people 40 years of age and older are also recommended.

Increasing and spreading modern ophthalmo-surgery.

Better training of and more eye doctors and paramedical personnel, increasing working facilities, transportation, working rooms, instruments and eye medicaments.

Above all:

1. Allocating a greater part of the national budget for public health activities;

2. Better cooperation between various branches of the government services, such as health, education, agriculture, social welfare and the like.

These are also much needed socio-ophthalmological activities on behalf of the blind.

ECONOMIC LOSS DUE TO BLINDNESS

Cost of Living	— RP. 60 milliard — US $ 144.5 million
Cost of Medical Treatment	— RP. 36 milliard — US $ 86.8 million
Loss of Productivity	— Rp. 36.16 milliard — US $ 92 million
TOTAL	Rp. 132.16 milliard — US $ 323.3 million

NUMBER OF EYE SPECIALISTS NEEDED

Now available	105
New eye doctors expected to complete their training every year	76

For the next 7 years, or by the year of 1981, there will be about 634 eye specialists.

For many years to come, each eye specialist will face a great number of demanding tasks.

BLINDNESS IN RURAL INDIAN CHILDREN

D.B. CHANDRA & P. KUMAR

(Allahabad, U.P. India)

In Allahabad located in North Central part of India, in 1973-74 a total of 74,620 persons had undergone visual screening; 1,548 blind persons were registered. The criteria for blindness were: 1). visual acuity not exceeding 3/60 in the better eye, 2). severe limitation of the field of vision to 20 degrees or less.

Blindness rate in this series came to 2,074 per hundred thousand of population.

Six and two-tenths percent of the totally blind were children. An estimate of the present adult blind population was made regarding the age at which they became blind. It was found that 125 (8.6%) were blind before the age of 15 years. Sixty-six (69.2%) of the blind children were from the rural areas.

The major causes of blindness were infections, nutritional deficiencies and accidents. Out of 66 blind children, 27 (40.9%) were curably blind and the rest, 39 (59.1%), were incurably blind. In these incurably blind patients, 33 (84.7%) cases were due to causes which could have been prevented. Thus only 9.09% of the existing blind patients were due to neither curable nor preventable causes.

Preventive measures such as mass education and prevention against nutritional deficiency diseases, vaccination against small pox, marriage counseling, ophthalmic screening of children, specialized ophthalmic school services, mobile ophthalmic services, measures for preventing needless eye injuries are presently used to reduce high numbers of needlessly blind patients.

BLINDNESS IN RURAL INDIAN CHILDREN

Since India is largely an agricultural country, 80% of its people live in rural areas. Hence, the larger percentage of blind are from rural populations.

A comparative review of blindness rate is presented from different countries: Canada, 131 blind persons per hundred thousand of population; U.S.A., 214 blind persons per hundred thousand of population; U.K., 200 blind persons per hundred thousand of population; India, 410 to 3.200 blind persons per hundred thousand of population.

Our study revealed 2,074 blind persons per hundred thousand of population.

There are regional variations of the causes of blindness in different parts of India. Conjunctival infections, including trachoma, are the major causes of blindness in children in the North, whereas keratomalacia takes the highest toll in West Bengal and the Southern States.

Our study was undertaken in the North-Central part of the country comprising the districts of Allahabad, Mirzapur and Pratapgarh. The criteria for blindness were: 1). visual acuity not exceeding 3/60, Snellen, in the better eye; 2). severe limitation of the field of vision not exceeding 20 degrees. The total population studied was 74,620. The total number of blind persons found was 1,548.

The blindness rate was 2,074 per hundred thousand population.

Adult Versus Child Blindness

	Children up to 15 Years of age	Adults	Total
Number	96	1,542	1,548
Percentage	6.20	93.80	100%

Ratio of Persons Who Developed Blindness in Childhood

	Developing Blindness in Childhood Before 15 Years of Age	Developed Blindness After 15 Years of Age	Total
Number	125	1,327	1,452
Percentage	8.6%	94.4%	100%

Rural Versus Urban Blindness in Children

	Rural	Urban	Total
Number	66	30	96
Percentage	69.2%	30.8%	100%

Etiology of Blindness in Rural Indian Children

Causes of Blindness	Type	Number	Percentage
Infection	Preventable	29	43.9
Malnutrition	Preventable	18	27.2
Accidents	Preventable	11	16.4
Congenital	Not preventable/ Preventable	3	4.3
Hereditary	Not preventable/ Preventable	3	4.3
Neoplasm	Not preventable	2	3.03
TOTAL		66	100%

Type of Blindness in Rural Indian Children

	Curable		Incurable	
	Preventable	Unpreventable	Preventable	Unpreventable
Number	17	10	33	6
Percentage	62.97	37.03	84.7	15.3
Number		27		39
Percentage		40.9		49.1

CONCLUSIONS:

1. In our series, 40.9 percent of blindness is curable.
2. Among 59.1% of incurable blindness 84.7% could have been prevented.
3. Only 9.09% of blindness was neither curable nor preventable.,

PREVENTIVE MEASURES:

There is an urgent need for continued governmental and public efforts for extensive preventive programs in rural areas of India with proper coordination between different agencies. To accomplish this need, mass education, improved sanitation, personal hygiene and the eradication of superstitions, bizzare beliefs, quack and home remedies is necessary. The use of pamphlets, exhibits, lectures, newspaper articles, film shows, radio and television are helpful in health education of the public.

Prevention of keratomalacia, malnutrition and diarrheas may be accomplished by distribution of dried skimmed milk fortified with Vitamin A or systemic administration of high doses of Vitamin A to children at risk, or distribution of foods rich in Beta Carotene to ill-fed populations.

Small pox may be prevented by vaccination. Marriage counseling may be of help. Screening of children for signs of deficiency and infectious eye diseases, vision testing in schools, the use of mobile ophthalmic services in rural areas and measures for preventing needless eye injuries by health education of the public are additional worthwhile measures in the prevention of blindness.

PREVENTION OF BLINDNESS THROUGH MOBILE
SURGERY IN RURAL AND URBAN AREAS IN PAKISTAN

T.H. KIRMANI

(Karachi, Pakistan)

Pakistan is a developing country. It has an agricultural economy. Eighty-five percent of its 70 million population lives in rural areas where socio-economic factors have great impact on the presence of disease, and particularly blindness.

Prevention of blindness is pursued through national and international agencies. The Royal Commonwealth Society for the Blind of the United Kingdom has played a particularly important role. It has assisted national agencies for more than a decade and has encouraged the establishment of Mobile Eye Service in 1968. In order to intensify prevention of blindness activities in Pakistan through Social Welfare Agencies, the Royal Commonwealth Society for the Blind initiated Mobile Eye Units in all parts of the country. Special emphasis was placed on work in rural areas where the need was particularly great.

Karachi is the largest city in Pakistan. In 1954 its population was 300,000. In 1974 it is nearly 4 million. This expansion of population has put great strain on the already meager available medical facilities. Overcrowding exists in the outpatient departments of hospitals. As many as 400 to 500 patients are examined daily. Poor people who live in the outskirts find it difficult to obtain treatment facilities for eye diseases. Some of them had to wait for four to five years before they could be admitted for needed eye surgery.

In Pakistan 85 percent of blindness is due to cararact and glaucoma. Both of these diseases are preventable and curable. The need was to provide Mobile Eye Hospital services. Such mobile surgical teams could visit the outskirts, examine and operate on patients in Mobile Operation Theaters under hospital conditions. This resulted in restoration of the vision of the needy and the poor who could not afford private care nor wait for long years. Amongst those are many bread-earners of families, who could not continue their work because of blindness. In order to rehabilitate them quickly, it was found necessary to arrange operation sessions in Mobile Eye Theaters close to their homes.

The technique of eye surgery for cataract and the requisite skill have been highly developed in Eastern countries. Cataract operations are successfully performed by skilled surgeons in a matter of ten minutes. Quick postoperative recovery within a week under careful supervision of medical and paramedical staff reduces the chances of complications to a minimum. Complications are fewer in eye camps than in the eye wards of the big

13

hospitals. The important factor for success of an eye camp is the skill of the surgeon, devotion to his work, and the cooperation of the community. In the outskirts of Karachi, 86 such eye camps have been successfully operating by the Mobile Eye Service of Pakistan since 1968. About 200,000 patients have been treated and over 15,000 operations for cataract and glaucome have been performed.

The standards of Mobile Surgical Teams have to be identical with those of surgical teams in big city hospitals. Use of cryosurgery helps to reduce post-operative cataract complications to a minimum. A good antibiotic cover is necessary. The incidence of infection, iris prolapse, and other complications are fewer because of extreme care taken by the Mobile Surgical Teams at these eye camps. The operation theater is set up in a large, airconditioned van. It has a facility of two operating tables and an area for sterilization, thus providing a high standard of surgical service.

Outpatient service is carried out every day throughout the week and round the year in the districts of Karachi. Over 100 patients are seen daily and patients are selected for surgery. This daily service also provides post-operative care. Whenever operative sessions are performed, the patiens' relatives act as nursing staff. They bring their own food along. This regular service and attendance by Mobile Surgical Teams create confidence in the work of the team. The reputation of the surgeon as the head of the surgical team is important in creating confidence in the patients. Regular attendance of the staff for follow-up is of equal importance. The blind are provided free operative facilities and eyeglasses by the Mobile Eye Service of Pakistan. Within a period of three to four weeks, the patients return to work happy to earn a livelihood for themselves and their dependents.

CAUSES, DIAGNOSIS AND PREVENTION OF BLINDNESS IN THE NORTH EAST DELTA REGION OF THE ARAB REPUBLIC OF EGYPT

M.H.M. EMARAH

(Mansoura, Egypt)

DEFINITION OF VISUAL IMPAIREMENT AND BLINDNESS

While each country defines blindness in relation to its social and economic standards, it is necessary to have a standard internationally accepted definition for blindness and another for visual impairement in order to compile international statistical data which attain a considerable degree of validity. As many as 65 definitions of blindness are listed in the report published in 1966 by the WHO. International surveys therefore are bound to be inaccurate.

In 1954, the World Assembly of the World Council for the Welfare of the Blind adopted the following definition of blindness and urged its acceptance as a minimum definition by all governments and organizations responsible for services of the blind:
1. Total absence of sight, or
2. Visual acuity not exeeding 3/60 or 10/200 (Snellen) in the better eye with correcting lenses, or
3. Serious limitations in the field of vision (generally not greater than 20 degrees).

The Council recognized that many persons with sight in the better eye, after correction, equal to 6/60 (or 20/200) are seriously handicapped visually, and it strongly urged that whenever possible the definition of blindness be expanded to include alle those with this degree of visual loss. However, this latter statement, though, may be theoretically feasible, yet in my opinion, we should differentiate in our statistical reports between two categories of visually handicapped persons, namely those who are totally blind and those who are partially sighted. This is because a patient with 6/60 vision is certainly capable to take care of his personal needs or maintain his social relations than a totally blind person. Therefore, it is here proposed to consider the problem of the visually handicapped patients under two main definitions.
1. A Totally Blind Person (T.B.P.): This denotes no perception of light in either eye.
2. A Partially Sighted Person (P.S.P.): This term applies to a person whose visual acuity does not exceed 6/60 in the better eye with correcting lenses, or a serious limitation in the field of vision not greater than 20 degrees.

15

CAUSES OF VISUAL IMPAIREMENT IN THE
NORTH EAST DELTA REGION OF THE A.R.E.

In an analysis of the records of 150000 patients who attended the Department of Ophthalmology of the University Hospital at Mansoura during the past five years, 772 patients were visually handicapped; 349 patients were males and 423 females. The incidence of visual incapacity in relation to age is given in Table I. The degree of visual incapacity is shown in Table II. The various causes of visual impairement, in order of frequency appears in Tables III and IV.

ACTIVITIES AIMED AT THE PRESERVATION OF SIGHT

The activities aimed at the preservation of sight in the Department of Ophthalmology of the University Hospital at Mansoura involve the following measures:
1. Screening all patients, over 30 years of age, who attend the outpatient and the refraction clinic for glaucoma. Treatment is commenced at an early stage before field changes of glaucomatous optic atrophy ensue.
2. Preventing and treating amblyopia in cases of strabismus. This is achieved by early surgical alignment of the visual axis in cases of tonic squint of early onset. In cases of accommodative squint, accurate correction of refractive error is done with occlusion of the good eye in cases of oveal fixation or pleoptics in cases with eccentric fixation.
3. Cataract is a major cause of curable blindness. Sight may be restored by cataract extraction. The operation is urged in intumescent cataract and in mature cataracts. Under no circumstance is a mature cataract neglected until it becomes hypermature. Bilateral congenital cataracts are treated as early as possible. The aspiration technique is the procedure of choice.
4. Prevention of diabetic retinopathy is achieved by routinely examining the members of the patient's family. Early control of diabetic retinopathy is of paramount importance. In addition to thorough medical control of the diabetes, fluorescein angiography is performed and any leaking blood vessels in the fundi are sealed by light coagulation.
It is of interest to note the rare incidence of diabetic retinopathy in patients with high myopia. Somehow, there may be a relationship between myopia and the delay on absence of retinopathy.
5. Study of the dominance of diseases known to have hereditary tendencies and furnishing advice to patients intending to marry from the same family.
6. Limiting the progression of blinding diseases such as trachoma by appropriate treatment at an early stage and improvement of sanitary conditions.
7. Restoring visual function in patients suffering from curable blindness, such as keratoplasty for corneal opacities.
8. Early diagnosis and treatment of retinal detachment. The fundi should be thoroughly examined in all patients attending for refraction.

TABLE I

Visual Incapacity in Relation to Age

Age	Number of Patients
I – Over 50 years	411
II – 25 – 50 years	212
III – 5 – 25 years	84
IV – Under 5 years	65
Total	772

TABLE II

Degree of Visual Incapacity

Degree of Visual Incapacity	Number of Eyes
I – N.P.L. (Totally Blind)	132
II – P.L.	72
III – H.M.	378
IV – C.F.--Less than some meter	276
V – Less than 6/60	786

TABLE III

Causes of Total Blindness in the Series (132 Eyes)

Cause	Number of Eyes
Glaucoma	45
Endophthalmitis	23
Trauma	18
Staphyloma	12
Uveitis	10
Detachment of Retina	8
Tumours	9
Diabetic Retinopathy	4
Vascular Occlusion	2
Optic Atrophy	1

17

TABLE IV

Causes of Visual Impairement (1412 Eyes)

Cause	Number of Eyes
Cataract	360
Glaucoma	236
Degenerative Myopia	198
Corneal Opacities	166
Diabetic Retinopathy	158
Retinal Detachment	134
Trauma	76
Uveitis	46
Retinitis Pigmentosa	16
Optic Atrophy	12
Vascular Occlusion	9
Heat Occupational Cataract	1

SUMMARY

A survey of the causes of blindness in the North East Delta Region of the Arab Republic of Egypt is given. Activities aimed at the preservation of sight are emphasized.

The author reports his observation of the rare incidence of diabetic retinopathy in highly myopic diabetic patients.

REFERENCES

Epidem. Vital Statist. 19: *437-511* (1966)
WHO Chronicle 21: *369-373* (1967)
WHO Chronicle 26: 28: (1972)
WHO Chronicle 27: *21-27* (1973)

REGISTRATION OF BLINDNESS IN SINGAPORE 1950-1972

KUANG HUI LIM

(Singapore)

In Singapore there is no national registration of persons with physical handicaps or blindness. An historical account may thus be traced of the practice and definition of blindness adopted in the country in order to study the pattern and problem of blindness locally. As far back as 1946, an attempt was made to maintain a count of blind persons by the Department of Health, now Ministry of Health. These early files were handed over to the Singapore Association for the Blind (S.A.B.) when it was founded in 1951 'to provide financial assistance and welfare for the blind.' It was not until 1953 that a register of blind persons was started. It was based on information provided by the government ophthalmologists at the then General Hospital. In 1953, Sir CLUTHA MACKENZIE, himself blind, was sent out by the Technical Assistance Administration of the United Nations, at the request of the Government of Singapore and the Federation of Malaya, to advise on a program for the blind, with particular reference to the development of blind services and facilities for rehabilitation. MACKENZIE's report (1953) contained an account given by the late Mr. A.D. WILLIAMSON, then eye surgeon at the General Hospital, on the chief sight destroying conditions prevailing at that time. They included keratomalacia, ophthalmia neonatorum, optic atrophy, cataract, congestive glaucoma, corneal ulceration, interstitial keratitis, iridocyclitis, penetrating wounds, intraocular tumours and trachoma. No actual figures were quoted.

DEFINITION OF BLINDNESS

Central visual acuity of 6/60 or worse with the best correcting lens, or a field defect in which the field has contracted to such an extent that the widest diameter of visual fields subtends an angular distance no greater than 20 degrees. Not specifically defined, it includes the less specific 'economic blindness which means inability to do any kind of work, industrial or otherwise, for which sight is essential.

In 1955, the Far East Conference on Work for the Blind met in Tokyo and recommended the recognition and implementation throughout the world the following definition: 'Total absence of sight, or visual acuity not exceeding 3/60 or 10/200 in the better eye with correcting lenses, or serious limitation in the field of vision, generally not greater than 20 degrees'.

The Government of the Federation of Malaya (Kuala Lumpur, 1956) accepted the definition of blindness as follows: 'a). Total absence of sight, and b). Visual acuity not exceeding 3/60 in the better eye with correcting lenses'.

REGISTRATION OF BLINDNESS IN SINGAPORE

Persons in Singapore were registered blind under two categories, viz: a). 'totally blind' of b). 'partially blind'. A person was certified 'totally blind' when he was unable to see anything, and 'partially blind' when he could make out movements and shadows but had insufficient eye-sight to carry on a occupation where vision was necessary. Monocular blindness, by definition, was not registered. Certification was carried out by the ophthalmologists at the General Hospital for the purpose of social aid and certification was not required by law. Blind persons who were not referred to the hospital were not registered.

PREVALENCE OF BLINDNESS

The yearly prevalence of blindness based on registration for the past 23 years shows a total of 1,959 registered and 517 deregistered persons between 1950-1972. The number of registered blind persons in Singapore on December 31, 1972, was 1,442, with a rate of 67 per 100,000 population. This compares unfavourably to the figure of 55 per 100,000 in 1964.

AGE AND SEX

The age and sex of registered blind persons in Singapore by 1970 shows a slight preponderance of males over females, with the largest majority of both sexes above 44 years of age.

CHANGING PATTERN OF BLINDNESS

A breakdown of blind persons registered according to cause for the 23-year-period from 1950-1972 revealed that congenital malformations were responsible for less than 10 percent prior to 1960. This figure increased to 15 percent in 1964, 15.4 percent in 1968 and 24 percent in 1972. There were acquired causes of blindness during the same period.

An analysis of 80 cases of congenital causes of blindness on the register in 1969 showed that of those born blind, the commonest causes were malformations (40 percent), congenital cataract (20 percent), optic atrophy (8 percent) and congenital glaucoma (5 percent).

Acquired causes of blindness for the past 23 years revealed glaucoma (28.6 percent) as the commonest cause. This was followed by optic atrophy (23.7 percent), corneal disease (18.5 percent) and retinal degeneration (9.6 percent). During 1965-1968 the acquired causes in order of frequency were glaucoma (26.6 percent), optic atrophy (25.9 percent), retinal degeneration (17.6 percent) and corneal disease (5.7 percent). During 1969-1972 the acquired causes were retinal disease (22 percent), glaucoma (20 percent), optic atrophy (20 percent) and corneal disease (12.3 percent).

LOCAL FACTORS AFFECTING THESE FINDINGS

A decline is seen in blindness due to infections and malnutrition. WILLIAMSON in 1953 observed that keratomalacia, ophthalmia neonatorum and optic atrophy were the major sight-destroying conditions at that time; LOH in 1964 reported the incidence of keratomalacia on the decline; by 1972, we could barely find a case of acute trachoma and xerophthalmia was virtually non-existent. These observations reflect improvements in the health of the citizens and the gains in the economy of the country.

PROSPECT FOR THE FUTURE IN SINGAPORE

Prospects for the future in Singapore are reflected in our prevention of blindness programs in terms of awareness of eye diseases that can cause blindness, safety precautions, adequate diagnosis, prompt treatment and research into causes of blindness.

According to Dr. ARTHUR LIM, 'Two factors are essential in any prevention of blindness program in a country. The first is awareness of the eye diseases that can cause blindness. This includes adequate training of medical personnel to recognize the blinding eye diseases. The second is preventive measures and treatment, based on education, built on research and directed towards the public in terms of educational campaigns, and, if necessary, backed up with measures for legislation.' Some succes in this direction has already been achieved in Singapore.

Research on ocular trauma, a common cause of loss of sight, is currently being pursued. It is hoped that data obtained will provide pointers for prevention, backed up if necessary with suggestions for legislation. As an example, eye injuries and blindness from firecrackers were totally eradicated when sale of fireworks was banned.

THE EARLY DETECTION OF GLAUCOMA

ERIK LINNÉR

(Goteborg, Sweden)

The International Ophthalmological Council has elected the following committee on the early detection of glaucoma consisting of: W. LEYDHECKER, Würzburg (BRD) (president) and the members M. ARMALY, Washington, D.C. (USA), E. LINNÉR, Umea, (Sweden), E.S. PERKINS, London, (Great Britain), TH. SCHMIDT, Bern, (Switzerland). The committee reviewed the present knowledge in the area of early detection of glaucoma and noted the following:

Glaucoma remains a major cause of blindness in all countries of the world. An undesirably large number of people are already blind from glaucoma in one or both eyes when they first seek the diagnostic help of the ophthalmologist. The group requiring most urgent attention is that where ocular hypertension has become associated with a typical defect in the visual field.

The development and progression of field defects result from the interaction of many factors the most important of which is increased ocular pressure level.

Progression of field defects can be arrested in the early stage by effective control of ocular pressure level; this desirable effect, however, becomes less achievable when the disease is in an advanced stage.

The incidence of glaucoma blindness increases significantly with age although it does not spare any age group; it occurs earlier in individuals with family history of glaucoma.

The risk to have or to develop glaucomatous defects increases with ocular pressure, age, family history of glaucoma, optic cup size and high myopia.

The committee concludes that the diagnosis and management of glaucoma remains the responsibility of the ophthalmologist only.

The early detection of glaucoma in the individual patient involves a careful ocular and general history, slit-lamp examination, tonometry, ophthalmoscopy and an examination of the visual field such as is possible only in the ophthalmologist office. Therefore in countries where ophthalmic care is available for the majority of the population, this system constitutes the ideal method of early detection. Ophthalmologists must seize this great opportunity to detect early glaucoma in every patient that seeks their diagnostic help.

A great effort must be made to increase the awareness of the public and the medical profession of the facts about glaucoma through a wide variety of programs of information and education.

The committee is aware that preventative ophthalmic care is not always

23

available to a large segment of the population in all countries and would recommend special public health effort where glaucoma detection programs are designed to maximally utilize the available manpower to best meet the health needs of the community, in concert with other preventative or detection health programs (x-rays mass screening, malnutrition, infection and cataract screening).

In order to best serve the interest of the patient, these programs must be under the professional direction of the ophthalmologist who can best decide on the selection of efficient and appropriate screening methods and coordinate their performance. Efficient screening methods include tonometry, ophthalmoscopy and visual field examination.

If non-medical personnel help in examinations for glaucoma detection they must understand their responsibility to refer suspected cases to an ophthalmologist.

Finally the committee wishes to highlight the fact that an important aspect of preventing glaucoma blindness is the selection of the appropriate therapeutic regimen, medical of surgical, that is realistic and practical for each patient.

GLAUCOMA BLINDNESS RATE IN BULGARIA

P. BANKOV & R. GOLEMINOVA

(Sofia, Bulgaria)

A statistical survey was done by ophthalmologists in 1970 in Bulgaria on blindness rate frequency.

It was found that there were 3312 blind persons in Bulgaria. This corresponded to 39 blind persons per 100,000 population. The criterion of blindness was visual acuity of the better seeing eye not better than 0.03 or 2/60.

Hereditary diseases led the list with 27.7 per cent; inflamatory diseases were second with 18.8 per cent; glaucoma was in third place causing 16.3 per cent of blindness.

541 persons were blind because of glaucoma. Expressed in percentages, 0.072 per cent of men and 0.056 per cent of women in Bulgaria were blind as a result of simple glaucoma. Life expectancy of women with glaucoma in Bulgaria is higher than that of men. This means that men become blind in Bulgaria more often than women.

The glaucoma blindness rate amongst the rural population is greater than that of the urban population. This correlation may be the result of medical attendance in the two groups of population. The glaucoma incidence rate in urban zones is about three times higher than that among rural population.

Approximately 15 per cent of the blind with glaucoma were less than 60 years old. The data showed 16.4 per cent of women and 13.3 per cent of men became blind before they were 50 years old.

Rheumatism was diagnosed in 5.9 per cent of the cases, diabetes 0.4 per cent and tuberculosis in 1.1 per cent.

Glaucomatous disease was diagnosed early in 13.0 per cent of the city dwellers and in 6.9 percent of the villagers.

The greater proportion of the blind were not operated upon. For instance, 56 percent of the glaucomatous blind eyes in cities and 62 percent of these eyes in villages did not undergo surgery. Those that did submit to surgery frequently postponed their operations until their vision became severely impaired. Residual vision of 0.03 resulted more often in operated cases than in not operated cases of glaucoma.

Acute congestive glaucoma occurred in 11.4 percent, chronic congestive glaucoma in 48.2 percent and simple glaucoma in 40.4 percent. The eyes that had acute congestive glaucoma ended up with poorer vision than those in the other two groups. This is believed to be due to delay in seeking treatment.

It appears that the prevalence of glaucoma blindness in Bulgaria is similar to that found in other countries. However, this does not mean that we must not exert continued efforts against preventing blindness caused by this disease. We must strive to further improve early diagnosis and treatment of glaucoma. We should also pay special attention to early surgery in acute congestive cases. The fear expressed by patients in Bulgaria regarding surgical intervention for glaucoma is unfounded.

PREVENTION OF HEREDITARY EYE DISEASE

IRENE HUSSELS MAUMENEE

(Baltimore, Maryland, U.S.A.)

During the past few decades, there has been in our clinic a relative increase of hereditary eye diseases compared to diseases of infectious or traumatic origin. A 1972 report from Montreal's Children's Hospital (SCRIBER, 1972) estimated that 30% of all pediatric admissions were the result of pure genetic diseases or diseases with strong genetic components. Similar proportions may well hold true for ophthalmology, though the actual percentage of genetic cases is not known.

What kind of disorders are we dealing with? Classically, autosomal dominant, recessive, and X-linked disorders are distinguished. Apart from this group, ocular malformations due to chromosomal aberrations and malformation syndromes, due to unknown etiology, have to be recognized. They might be of polygenic or multi-factorial inheritance; they can be the result of interaction of several genes, or of one or more genes plus environmental influence, or be solely caused by intrauterine infections. The specific disorders have recently been reviewed (HUSSELS-MAUMENEE, 1974).

AUTOSOMAL DOMINANT INHERITANCE

Let us first consider the classic patterns of single-locus multipleallele inheritance. Autosomes are present in pairs. One autosome is paternally derived and the other is maternally derived. Females have paired X chromosomes, one paternal and one maternal, whereas males have a paternal Y and maternal X chromosome. Thus, at a given locus any person carries two alleles and is said to be homozygous for a given gene if the two alleles are identical. He is said to be *heterozygous* if the two alleles are different. A male is called *hemizygous* with regard to genes carried on the X chromosome, since the Y chromosome seems genetically inactive except for sex-determining genes and does not provide genes complementary to the X chromosome. A gene is said to be *dominant* if it is manifest in the heterozygous state. It is called *recessive* if it has to be homozygous in order to be evident clinically.

Autosomal dominant inheritance is safely established if there is transmission through at least three generations and if father and son are affected in consecutive generations. Father-to-son transmission excludes *X-linked inheritance*, which can very closely simulate autosomal dominant inheritance.

The author is supported by Research Career Development Award GM 70124 from the National Institutes of Health, Education, and Welfare.

However, an X-linked trait never can be transmitted from an affected father to his son, because a father gives only his Y chromosome to his male offspring, never his X chromosome (which carries the X-linked trait).

In many instances it is safe to change the criterion of dominance from three to two generations. However, this is impossible in an inbred population, as represented by any racial or religious group which shows frequent intermarriage. It then can happen that a homozygously affected individual marries a heterozygous carrier of the trait and thus has 50 percent affected offspring. This so-called *pseudodominance* is frequently observed in relatively common diseases, such as retinitis pigmentosa.

On the average, 50 percent of the children of an affected person are affected; by chance there may be a high variability in the number of affected individuals in a given family. Dominant diseases affect both sexes in equal proportions, although the sex distribution can by chance deviate in a small family. Offspring of a healthy person do not run any risk of disease, except if the *penetrance* is reduced. This may lead to skipped generations, as occurs in retinoblastoma, or apparently skipped generations, due to the fact that the disease is so mild in a given person that it is not detectable by ordinary means. This is observed in many of the dominant diseases, such as the Marfan or von Hippel-Lindau syndrome.

A common cause for 'reduced penetrance' is delayed age of onset. A clinically healthy but carrier person may die after having children but before manifesting the disease. The children later develop the same disorder that affected their grandparents. Delayed age of onset is common in Huntington's chorea and myotonic dystrophy.

AUTOSOMAL RECESSIVE INHERITANCE

The minimal sufficient criterion for diagnosis of recessive inheritance is the presence of an identical disease in two sibs whose parents are normal. Several criteria strengthen this diagnosis. The most important is the detection of an enzymatic defect. If there is no female affected, neither of these two criteria is sufficient, however, since enzyme defects are also commonly at the basis of X-linked recessive disorders.

Consanguinity — that is, identity by descent — is commonly observed among parents of children with a rare recessive disorder. This is due to the fact that people who have one or more ancestors in common are more likely to carry one and the same deleterious gene and to give it to their common offspring. This occurs in one-quarter of the children of parents who carry one gene in common. Two-quarters of one-half of their children are heterozygous carriers and one-quarter of their children are perfectly normal phenotypically and genetically. Both sexes are equally affected. Heterozygosity of the parents is detected as a rule, because they have one or more affected children. The diagnosis is not made in those families in which all children are normal.

X-LINKED INHERITANCE

X-linked inheritance was first described for color blindness and became widely publicized with the occurrence of hemophilia in the European royal families. The defective or mutant gene is carried on the X chromosome and is thus transmitted from carrier mother to half of her sons. One-half of her daughters will be carriers. Sons who receive the defective gene will manifest the disease, since they are hemizygous for it; that is, they do not carry a corresponding healthy gene on their Y chromosome.

Females carrying two affected X's will show the disease to the same extent as the affected males. This phenomenon, which has been observed for mild and common disorders such as color blindness, can occur only if an affected man marries a carrier woman.

Another way for a woman to manifest the disease is through unfortunate *lyonization*. MARY LYON was the first to develop a hypothesis about the occasional severe manifestations of an X-linked disorder in heterozygous carrier women. Around the sixteenth day of embryogenesis, inactivation of one of the two X chromosomes occurs in all female embryonic cells with the exception of the gonadal cells. The inactivated X chromosome can be demonstrated as a Barr body in the buccal smear, for example, or in drumsticks of peripheral segmented leukocytes. On the average, 50 percent of the paternal X's and 50 percent of the maternal X's are inactivated. However, this number can vary considerably by chance, and it is certainly possible that all the X chromosomes of one of the parents might be inactivated. If the healthy chromosome is inactivated, and the X chromosome from the other parent carries a mutant gene, the full disease picture can arise in a female. Very high degrees of factor VIII deficiency, for example, have been observed in women.

Female carriers for several diseases can be detected, depending upon degree of sophistication of the examiner and the sensitivity of the laboratory techniques. In X-linked disorders for which no enzyme defect has been found, prenatal sex diagnosis is possible by amniocentesis, and abortion of males can be performed. This is a very inefficient method, since one-half of the aborted males are normal, and one-half of the living girls are carriers.

CHROMOSOMAL ABERRATIONS

TJIO & LEVAN in 1956, established that the normal chromosome complement of humans is 46 and not 48 as was previously thought. In the following years, multiple chromosomal diseases were delineated; that is, the correlation of previously idiopathic diseases with chromosomal aberrations was made. Numerical of structural abnormalities of the gonosomes, that is the X- and Y-chromosomes, are not accompanied by ocular findings per se, but change the laws usually applicable to X-chromosomal inheritance. An XXY male, having the Klinefelter syndrome, might not show the full blown symptomatology of an X-linked disorder as expected to be found in the male, but might show the mitigated form characteristic of the female carrier. Conversely, an XO Turner girl will be fully affected with an X-linked disorder since she is hemizygous for the X chromosome as is the rule for males. Chromosomal aberrations characteristically showing ocular findings are trisomies 13, 18, and 21, the deletion syndromes: 4p-(Wolf syndrome), 5p-(Cri-du-chat syndrome), 13q- and 18q-.

In addition a number of syndromes are well delineated clinically for which the etiologic agent is unknown. No evidence for Mendelian inheritance can be detected in them, nor has a chromosomal deletion been found up to this point. However, it may be suggested that at least some of them are due to minute deletions which, as of now, are not detectable by light miscroscopy.

I mention two examples: the Cornelia de Lange syndrome presented here in a Negro child and the Goldenharr syndrome as seen in a young girl who has the characteristic epibulbary dermoid, the upper lid coloboma and the preauricular appendages.

THERAPY OF GENETIC DISEASES

What can be done? Therapy of genetic diseases was, for a long time, approached symptomatically; thus, surgery for congenital cataracts was performed, dislocated lenses were extracted in patients with the Weill-Marchesani or Marfan syndromes. In recent times, therapy of inborn errors of metabolism has been attempted by various means; one being dietary control, as used in galactosemia, homocystinuria, and Refsum disease, to mention only a few; or chelation of excessive metabolities as applied to Wilson's disease where decreased levels of ceruloplasmin result in poor transport of free Cu_{2+} ions and storage of copper in tissues such as brain, liver, and cornea. The resulting clinical signs are basal ganglia degeneration, liver cirrhosis and the Kayer-Fleischer ring. However, these clinical signs revert partially or totally after the administration of D-penicillamine, a chelator of copper ions at the tissue level. Replacement of the deficient enzyme has been attempted for the mucopolysaccharidoses with only partial clinical succes. Some success was noticed in Fabry's disease but not in Tay Sachs disease.

By increasing the coenzyme of specific enzymatic reactions, the metabolic rate may be sufficiently raised to result in partial reversal of chemical signs. Thus in patients with homocystinuaria who are receiving vitamin B6 therapy, the urine may be cleared of homocystin, and there may be at least an arrest of this progressive degenerative disorder.

The foregoing approaches to therapy are still in their early stages. Therefore, in this disease group, more than in other diseases, prevention of birth of affected children is the goal. This may be done at several levels. Classically genetic counseling is given to families at risk; however, families at risk are usually detected after the birth of at least one affected child. In recent years, increasing efforts have been made to identify heterozygous carriers prior to the first pregnancy. Several prerequisites for population screening have consequently been defined. Precise biochemical diagnostic tests are needed to separate homozygous affected from heterozygous carriers and heterozygous carriers from the low normal homozygous people. It seems ethical that screening of the population should only be done once the screener has something to offer; that is, prenatal diagnosis, not only genetic counseling. To plan and organize such service of populations, community

30

education is of prime importance. Prenatal diagnosis of chromosomal aberrations and of an increasing number of inborn errors of metabolism and of dominant disorders is possible. Indications for amniocentesis may be apparent only after taking the family history, examination of autopsy reports, photographs of previously born and possibly dead children with respect to chromosomal aberrations and heterozygous manifestations. The patient is told to return between the 14th and 16th week of pregnancy. At that time, the position of the placenta is determined by ultrasound. This also permits the detection of a twin pregnancy. Thereafter, amniocentesis is performed using a transabdominal approach under local anesthesia. The technique consists of inserting a spinal needle through the midline of the abdominal wall and directing it towards the center of the uterine cavity. After entry into the uterus, the stylet is removed and 10 to 20 milliliters of amniotic fluid is aspirated. It is replaced in less than three hours. Amniotic fluid cells are quite pleomorphic immediately after amniocentesis. Over days of culture this changes with the disappearance of large polygonial cells and the progressive growth of other cells that resemble cultured fibroblasts. The amniotic fluid cells are of fetal origin and are derived mainly from fetal skin and amnion.

Many enzymes are present in amniotic fluid. They may be absent in specific inborn errors of metabolism. For example, hexosaminidase deficiency in amniotic fluid may be diagnostic of Tay-Sachs disease and glucosidase deficiency of Pompe's disease. It appears that dermatan sulfate is normally present in amniotic fluids while heparan sulfate is normally absent. Based upon this observation, is has been possible to diagnose Hurler or Hunter syndrome in utero using the presence of excess dermatan sulfate and the presence of heparan sulfate to prove the diagnosis. There is still great hesitation in using amniotic fluid alone for diagnostic enzyme assays without confirmation of the defect in cultured amniotic fluid cells. This caution presently extends to almost all hereditary biochemical disorders.

Amniotic fluid cells are then cultured. Cultivation is much more successful in early than in late pregnancy. The total number of cells in amniotic fluid rises steeply between the 20th and 25 th week of gestation, but the number of vital cells increases only slightly during this period. About 10% of amniotic fluid samples are grossly bloody and microscopic evidence of erythrocyte contamination can be found in most samples. Excess red blood cells may inhibit the rate of growth of the amniotic fluid cells and should be removed. Blood-free amniotic fluid samples are centrifuged at 1,200 r.p.m. for 15 minutes to remove the supernatant which is stored frozen. The cell pellate is re-suspended in Eagle minimum essential medium with 15% fetal calf serum added. Aliquots are placed in four to eight Petri dishes at 37° Celsius in an atmosphere of 5% CO_2 and air. The cells which have not attached to the Petri dish are removed after 24 hours. After 10 to 21 days in culture with feeding twice weekly, there are usually sufficient colonies of cells for passage with .25% trypsin into dishes containing glass cover slips. These cells are allowed to attach and grow for 24 hours after which colcemide is added to medium and the chromosome analysis is performed as previously described. Cells that are grown for biochemical studies for prenatal determination of an inborn error of metabolism are passaged repeatedly until sufficient cells are obtained for the planned specific chemical assay. When the assay results are available, no further cells are required for repeat studies. Then in addition the karyotype is determined as described earlier. The karyotype is routinely performed in cases where an amniocentesis was done to exclude an inborn error of metabolism. The opposite is not true if there is no specific indication for search of an abnormality.

Indications for amniocentesis are thus chromosomal abnormalities in the form of translocation carriers, advanced maternal age, previous child with Down syndrome, or with another chromosomal abnormality. AUBREY MILUNSKY in his recent book: Prenatal Diagnosis of Hereditary Disorders, published by Charles C. Thomas in 1973, undertook a questionnaire survey of the U.S. and Canadian experiences with amniocentesis for prenatal genetic studies. A total of 1,663 cases were collated of which 1,368 were done to exclude chromosomal disorders; 115 in order to determine the sex because of an X-linked disorder; and 180 to rule out an inborn error of metabolism. Among 1,368 amniocenteses that were performed for chromosomal disorders, abnormalities were detected in 36 fetuses. The diagnosis was confirmed in all cases where the outcome was known. The fetal sex was incorrectly diagnosed in 7 out of 1,663 cases. In all these cases, males were born instead of the predicted female infants. No instance was the fetal sex incorrectly diagnosed where an X-linked disorder was to be ruled out. Also in one instance, galactosemia was diagnosed in a child whereas the infant was normal and one diagnosis of a normal fetus was made and the child had the Hurler syndrome. One fetus with polyploidy in cultured amniotic fluid cells was aborted before it was well established that polyploidy is a normal feature of amniotic fluid cells culture. The child was also normal.

Complications after amniocentesis may be viewed in three groups: that is early, meaning within two weeks after amniocentesis; intermediate, meaning within more than to weeks after amniocentesis; and late in the third trimester. In the above mentioned, 1,663 amniocenteses, early complications occurred in 19 cases, giving an early complication rate of about 1%. But not all of these complications can be related to the procedure since a certain number of abortions are expected to occur spontaneously around those weeks. There were 6 cases of short-term vaginal bleeding which resulted in normal infants, three cases of abortion; two cases of vaginal bleeding followed by an abortion. In the group of intermediate complications, 16 cases of abortions were noted. A total of 36 fetuses were lost out of 1,663 children, which gives a complication rate of about 2%, which is including all cases which would have aborted spontaneously and where fetal deaths would have occured because of severe malformations. Thus, fetal deaths may result from rupture of the placenta, amnionitis, fetal hemorrhage and puncture of the fetus, as evidenced by the case described by CROSS & MAUMENEE, 1973. These risks for the fetus have to be weighed against the disease risk for which amniocentesis is being performed in the first place.

Among the X-linked disorders, which may present an indication for amniocentesis and prenatal diagnosis, several are relevant to the ophthalmologist (Table I): choroideremia and X-linked retinitis pigmentosa; Fabry's disease; Lowe's oculo-cerebro-renal syndrome; and Norrie's disease, as well as mucopolysaccharidosis type II or Hunter's syndrome. Several others can probably come to the mind of the scrutinizer. In Fabry's and Hunter's disease, the affected male fetus can be clearly distinguished from the unaffected male fetus. Cultivated amniotic fluid cells can be stained for the sex body or Barr body (Feulgen). The overall accuracy of this method of sex diagnosis is about 95%. Also Y-chromosome fluorescence after staining with quinacrine mustard can be used simultaneously. It is wise to always do a full karyotype as well. Amniocentesis is indicated in the following recessive metabolic diseases with eye involvement (Table 2).

Thus in summary, classical genetic counseling is no longer the only tool of the geneticist, but population screenings, prenatal diagnosis and the first attemps to treatment have been successfully undertaken.

TABLE I

X-linked syndromes for which prenatal sex diagnosis may be indicated

1. Choroideremia
2. Fabry disease
3. Mucopolysaccharidosis type II Hunter
4. Norrie disease
5. Ocular albinism
6. Oculo-cerebro-renal syndrome of Lowe
7. Retinitis pigmentosa

TABLE II

Selected inborn errors of metabolism for which prenatal diagnosis is possible

1. Sandhoff disease
2. Tay-Sachs disease
3. Generalized gangliosidosis
4. Mucopolysaccharidoses
5. Refsum disease
6. Cystinosis
7. Homocystinuria
8. Galactosemia

REFERENCES

HUSSELS-MAUMENEE, I. Genetic counseling in: Genetic and Metabolic Eye Disease. M.F. Glodberg, ed., Little Brown and Co. Boston, Massachusetts, 1974.
MILUNSKY, A. The Prenatal diagnosis of Hereditary Disorders. C.C. Thomas Publishers, Springfield, Illinois, 1973.
SCRIBER, C. Pers. comm., Bar Harbor, (1972).
TJIO, I.H. & LEVAN, A. The chromosome number of man. *Hereditas* 42: *1*, (1956).

METABOLIC EYE DISEASE DIAGNOSABLE
BY AMNIOCENTESIS

E.R. BERMAN & S. MERIN

(Jerusalem, Israel)

It is a credit to the organizers of this meeting that the subject of 'Amniocentesis in the prevention of blindness' has been included in the program. The rapidly growing body of information in this field has only recently been brought to the attention of ophthalmologists (MILUNSKY, 1974). There are presently four groups of genetically caused diseases leading to impaired vision or to blindness that are amenable to prevention by amniocentesis. Before discussing them, however, certain general comments about amniocentesis should be made.

The story of amniocentesis started in the early 1960's with the discovery by RIIS & FUCHS 1960 that sex chromatin analyses can be made on amniotic fluid. Today, amniocentesis is accepted everywhere as a simple and well established method for providing rich and valuable information about the future baby. This has been made possible by major technical advances in both the amniocentesis technique itself (NADLER & GERBIE, 1970) and in tissue culture methodology. In addition, the elucidation of the enzymatic basis of many hereditary diseases, as well as the establishment of karyogenetics (or cytogenetics), completes the list of tools necessary for the prevention of these diseases.

Amniocentesis is usually performed between the 15th and 18th week of pregnancy and may be done in the outpatient clinic. Provided it is performed by qualified obstetricians, the risk of complications today is considered to be very low (DANCIS, 1973; HOWELL, 1973). Nevertheless complications may occur, such as those described recently by CROSS, & MAUMENEE (1973). This was an unusual case of severe ocular trauma during amniocentesis, manifesting as a congenital epithelial cyst of the anterior chamber. To data more than 1,000 amniocenteses have been carried out to monitor pregnancies at risk for genetic diseases, and cytological or biochemical data are available on at least half of them.

We have grouped into four categories those genetic disorders leading to impaired vision or to blindness which can be prevented by amniocentesis. Considered in order of feasibility and reliability, as well as statistical data presently available, these consist of: biochemical defects or inborn errors of metabolism, x-linked disorders, morphological abnormalities and chromosomal anomalies.

Amniocentesis is theoretically possible in any disorder whose enzymatic defect has been established. This applies particularly to the inborn errors of metabolism. Nearly one hundred genetically determined metabolic disorders have been delineated in recent years. However, only some of them have ocular manifestations, and not all are amenable to diagnosis by amniocentesis. In reviewing the literature, and taking into account our own experience as well, there are now about twenty metabolic eye diseases that are diagnosable by amniocentesis. In roughly half of them, amniocentesis has already been performed, and in the remainder, amniocentesis is theoretically possible but has not yet been reported — to the best of our knowledge — probably for technical reasons only.

A word of caution about the use of cultured versus uncultured cells for performing enzyme studies: The number of viable cells in any amniotic fluid sample is highly variable, and although enzymes are present, their specific activities — when based on parameters such as protein or DNA content — are highly erratic. When the relative content of a specific component has to be precisely determined (as for instance in Tay-Sachs disease) then the use of uncultured cells may give rise to serious diagnostic errors. Therefore, culturing of cells, even though causing a delay of 4 to 6 weeks, is highly recommended by most investigators.

Tables 1 and 2 summarize the genetic disorders, their main ocular signs and the enzymatic or biochemical defects that form the basis of the various tests performed on the amniotic cells. Tay-Sachs disease has been placed first on the list for many reasons, the foremost being that it has now become the prototype of all genetic disorders. The first clinical description of this disease came before the turn of the century, and through the efforts of many investigators over the years, we now understand the mode of transmission, the chemistry of the storage substances and the nature of the enzymatic defect.

The deficiency of a specific enzyme, hexosaminidase A, leads to the accumulation of G_{M2}-ganglioside (Fig. 1) and its asialo derivative in the brain and in the ganglionic cell layer of the retina at levels 300 times greater than normal. It is this accumulation that causes both cellular destruction (clinically manifested by the cherry red spot and blindness) and the neurological changes that characterize this fatal disorder. Tay-Sachs disease is transmitted by an autosomal recessive gene and is much more common in certain Jewish communities, which provide the main population at risk.

Credit for elucidating the enzymatic deficiency is given to Dr JOHN S. O'BRIEN and his colleagues at the University of California OKADA & O'BRIEN, 1969). Their discovery not only led to effective means for diagnosing affected indivuduals, but also for detecting heterozygotes. More recently the enzyme assay has provided the basis for monitoring pregnancies in high risk individuals, i.e. women who have already given birth to one affected child, or women known to be heterozygotes (O'BRIEN, 1973).

We have summarized the results of amniocentesis reported from four of the leading centers now doing this as a routine procedure for all pregnancies at risk. Over 100 amniocenteses have been performed throughout the world (Table 3) and the results are extremely encouraging. The largest number of diagnoses have been made at the Sheba Medical Center in Tel Aviv, where patients are referred from all over Israel. Out of 28 cases predicted to be homozygous for Tay-Sachs disease at the four centers listed, all but one were aborted in time and the diagnosis confirmed. Only one case was un-

TABLE I

Metabolic eye disorders – Amniocentesis performed

Disorder	Ocular signs	Enzymatic or biochemical defect
G_{M2}-gangliosidosis Type I (Tay-Sachs)	Cherry red spot in macula	Hexosaminidase A
Hurler syndrome (MPS I-H)	Corneal clouding. Retinal degeneration	α-L-Iduronidase
*Hunter syndrome (MPS II)	Retinal degeneration	Sulfoiduronate sulfatase
G_{M1}-gangliosidosis Type I (generalized) gangliosidosis)	Cherry red spot in macula (50% of cases). Corneal clouding (some cases)	β-galactosidase
*Fabry's disease	Corneal whorl. Vascular changes	Ceramide α-galactosidase
Niemann-Pick	Cherry red spot in macula	Sphingomyelinase
Cystinosis, infantile	Crystals in cornea and conjunctiva. Pigmentary retinopathy	Storage of cystine
G_{M2}-gangliosidosis Type II (Sandhoff's disease)	Cherry red spot in macula	Hexosaminidase A and B
Krabbe's disease	Optic atrophy	Cerebroside β-galactosidase
**I-cell disease	Corneal clouding	Defective lysosomal enzymes

*   Also detectable as an x-linked syndrome.
** May also be diagnosed by morphological abnormalities.

successful because the amniocentesis was performed too late for a safe abortion. The child was born and subsequently developed the disorder. We can say that by mass screening of high risk populations, i.e. Jews of Ashkenazi origin, to detect the carriers, and by monitoring the pregnancies of known heterozygotes, the tools are now in our hands to control this tragic disease.

Of the mucopolysaccharidoses (Table 1), the specific enzymatic defects in both Huler's and Hunter's syndromes are now known. Amniocentesis has also been performed to detect other rare diseases (Table 1) of which two, G_{M1}-gangliosidosis Type I and Niemann-Pick disease, are fatal in the first years of life. The clinical pictures are well known to us and their enzymatic defects are deficiencies of B-galactosidase and sphingomyelinase, respectively.

TABLE II

Metabolic eye disorders – Amniocentesis possible

Disorder	Ocular signs	Enzymatic or biochemical defect
Galactosemia	Cataract	Galactose-1-phos. uridyl transferase
Metachromatic leukodystrophy	Grayness of macula	Arylsulfatase A
Refsum's syndrome	Pigmentary degeneration	Phytanic acid oxidase
Galactokinase deficiency	Cataract	Galactokinase
Homocystinuria	Lens dislocation	Cystethionine synthase
Maple syrup urine disease	Ptosis; nystagmus; strabismus	Decarboxylation of 3 branched-chain keto acids
Hyperlysinemia	Lens dislocation	Lysine metabolism
*Pseudo-Hurler polydystrophy (ML III)	Corneal clouding	Defective lysosomal enzymes
Xeroderma pigmentosa	Squamous cell carcinomas of lids	DNA endonuclease

* May also be diagnosed by morphological abnormalities

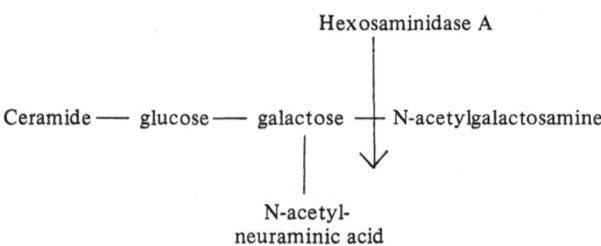

Fig. 1. Tach-Sachs disease, G_{M2} gangliosidosis Type 1.

Four other disorders shown in Table I complete the list of diseases in which amniocentesis has already been performed and diagnosis made on the basis of specific biochemical defects. In cystinosis, large amounts of the amino acid cystine are found; in G_{m2}-gangliosidoses type II, both hexosaminidase A and B are deficient; in Krabbe's disease a deficiency of cerebroside-B-galactosidase leads to excess storage of lipids in the optic

TABLE III

Prenatal diagnosis of Tay-Sachs disease

| | Number of fetuses | | | |
Number of pregnancies monitored	Predicted to be affected	Confirmed to be affected	Author, year, location	Reference number
44	10	10	NAVON, 1974, Tel Aviv	(10)
32	8	7	O'BRIEN, 1973, California	(8)
17	7	7	SAIFER et al., 1973, New York	(11)
10	3	3	ELLIS et al., 1973, London	(12)
Total 103	28	27		

nerve; and in I-cell disease, one of the mucolipidoses, there is a generalized deficiency of lysosomal enzymes.

In the disorders listed in Table 2, amniocentesis has not yet been performed but is theoretically possible since the enzyme defect has been established. It is only a question of time before these disorders may also be brought under control.

We should now like to turn to another group of genetic disorders also preventable by amniocentesis, namely those transmitted as x-linked recessive traits (Table 4). Some of the disorders shown in this table are con-

TABLE IV

X-linked eye disorders detectable by prenatal determination of sex

Localized
      Choroidemia
      x-linked albinism
      x-linked retinitis pigmentosa
      x-linked retinoschisis

Systemic
      Norrie's disease
      Hunter's syndrome
      Fabry's disease
      Lowe's syndrome

fined to the eye, and determining the sex of the fetus provides the only way for considering a therapeutic abortion. In families where the mother is known to be a carrier, future pregnancies should be monitored. In the fetal sex is found to be a female, the pregnancy is not terminated. But if it is a male, then there is a 50 per cent chance that he will be affected and abortion seems justified.

Other disorders listed in Table 4 are systemic in nature. Of these, Hunter's syndrome and Fabry's disease can be diagnosed by means of the specific enzymatic defect in addition to the sex determination, and so provide a 100 per cent prediction of the disease instead of only 50 per cent prediction.

39

While still on the subject of metabolic disorders, we would like to discuss another parameter that may be used diagnostically in prenatal diagnoses. The parameter is morphology, i.e. examination of cultured amniotic cells by electron microscopy. This may be of use in a recently described group of disorders termed mucolipidoses, of which some are listed in Table 5. These

TABLE V

Amniocentesis and the mucolipidoses

Diagnosis possible by enzyme assay
    Fucosidosis
    Mannosidosis
    Mucolipidosis II (I-cell disease)
    Mucolipidosis III

Diagnosis possible by electron microscopy
    Mucolipidosis I
    Mucolipidosis IV

---

syndromes are classified together because they are storage diseases in which both lipids and complex carbohydrates (either mucopolysaccharides or glycoproteins) accumulate within the cell. The abnormal morphology is most readily detected in cells obtained either from liver or conjunctival biopsy, or from cultured skin fibroblasts. Single membrane limited vacuoles are thought to represent lysosomes distented by excess storage of mucopolysaccharides, while the lamellar bodies probably represent stored lipids (Fig. 2).

In the last two disorders listed in Table 5, no obvious biochemical or enzymatic abnormality has as yet been detected. In the condition that we have termed mucolipidosis IV (BERMAN et al, 1974), corneal clouding is a very early finding. We are presently studying three infants in Israel originating from 3 different families who seem to have this syndrome. In Fall of 1973 one of the mothers became pregnant, and came to us for counseling. Amniocentesis was performed and the cells successfully cultured; however examination by electron microscopy did not reveal any abnormal storage bodies. The child subsequently born appears — for the present at least — to be unaffected.

To complete the picture of ocular disorders which can be prenatally detected by amniocentesis, chromosomal abnormalities may also be included (Table 6). It should, however, be recalled that chromosomal anomalies, in contrast to the three previous groups, are not, strictly speaking, hereditary diseases. So, with the exception of Down's syndrome, the population-at-risk cannot be known. In this disorder the relationship between maternal age and familial translocations may indicate the high-risk populations among pregnant women. The other chromosomal anomalies can hardly be detected because of their sporadic appearance, unless mass screenings are performed.

In the chromosomal anomalies shown in Table 6, the ocular manifestations of the disease are always accompanied by varying degrees of systemic manifestations such as cardiovascular, skeletal, neurological and facial ab-

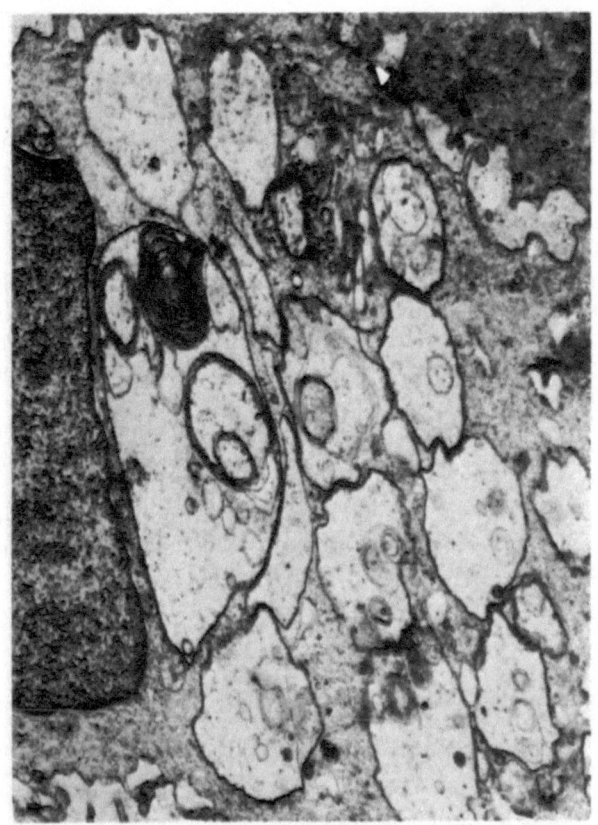

Fig. 2. Electron micrograph of a conjunctival fibroblast from a new mucolipidosis variant (ML IV).

TABLE VI

Chromosomal abnormalities

Syndrome	Abnormality	Ocular manifestations
Patau's	Trisomy 13	Coloboma, retinal dysplasia, microphthalmus
Edward's	Trisomy 18	Abnormal palpebral fissure, ptosis, squint
Down's	Trisomy 21	Abnormal palpebral fissure, Brushfield spots, squint, cataract, blepharitis
Cri-du-chat	$5p^-$	Hypertelorism
	$18q^-$, $18p^-$, $18r$	Various anomalies

41

normalities. In Patau's syndrome retinal dysplasia is a common finding and the patient is usually blind from birth. In all the other chromosomal anomalies the eyes are usually less severely affected.

As yet there is no possibility of detecting the most common genetically-caused blinding disease, retinitis pigmentosa. Despite all the efforts made over the years, we still do not know the basic enzymatic or biochemical defect that causes the visual cell degeneration. As the typical recessively inherited retinitis pigmentosa is a localized disorder, the changes of finding an enzymatic or biochemical abnormality in other cells in the body, such as the skin, are unlikely. The same is true of infantile and juvenile heredomacular dystrophies, a major cause of visual impairement in young people. There is also, as yet, no indication that the more common hereditary corneal dystrophies, the hereditary congenital cataracts or most of the congenital glaucomas have a detectable systemic abnormality.

To conclude, we would like to point out that amniocentesis provides a new and powerful tool to combat a group of diseases which were almost unpreventable till now, the hereditary diseases of the eye. This is especially important in view of the fact that hereditary diseases of the eye have become a relatively common cause of blindness in childhood, and that in most cases they are untreatable.

REFERENCES

BERMAN, E.R., LIVNI, N., SHAPIRA, E., MERIN, S. & LEVIJ I.S. Congenital corneal clouding with abnormal systemic storage bodies: a new variant of mucolipidosis. *J. Pediat.*, 84: *519* (1974).

CROSS, H.E. & MAUMENEE, A.E. Ocular trauma during amniocentesis. *Arch. Ophthal.*, 90: *303* (1973).

DANCIS, J. The prenatal detection of hereditary defects, in: Medical Genetics, Ed. by V.A. McKusick & R. Clairborne, HB Publishing Co., Inc., New York, p. 247, 1973.

ELLIS, R.B., IKONNE, J.U., PATRICK, A.D., STEPHENS, R. & WILLCOX, P. Prenatal diagnosis of Tay-Sachs disease. *Lancet* II: *1144* (1973).

HOWELL, R.R. Prenatal diagnosis in the prevention of handicapping disorders. *Pediat. Clin. North America* 20: *141* (1973).

MILUNSKY, A. Hereditary eye disease and prenatal diagnosis. *Arch. Ophthal.*, 91: *169* (1974).

NADLER, H.L. & GERBIE, A.B. Role of amniocentesis in intrauterine detection of genetic disorders. *New Engl. J. Med.*, 282: *596* (1970).

NAVON, R. Personal communication (1974).

O'BRIEN, J.S. Tay-Sachs disease: from enzyme to prevention. *Fed. Proc.*, 32: *191* (1973).

OKADA, S. & O'BRIEN, J.S. Tay-Sachs disease: generalized absence of a beta-D-N-acetylhexosaminidase component. *Science*, 165: *698* (1969).

RIIS, P. & FUCHS, F. Antenatal determination of fetal sex in prevention of hereditary diseases. *Lancet* II: *180* (1960).

SAIFER, A., SCHNECK, L., PERLE, G., VALENTI, C. & VOLK, B.W. Caveats of antenatal diagnosis of Tay-Sachs disease. *Amer. J. Obs. & Gynec.*, 115: *553* (1973).

HOMOCYSTINURIA

J. FRANÇOIS

(Ghent, Belgium)

Homocystinuaria was first described by FIELD and his co-workers. It is an inborn error of sulphur amino acid — methionine — metabolism. It is caused by the absence or deficiency of cystathionine synthase which normally transforms homocysteine and serine in cystathionine in the liver and brain. As a result of the lack of this enzyme methionine, homocysteine and homocystine accumulate in the plasma cerebrosphinal fluid and tissues, while homocystine and homocysteine are also excreted in the urine up to 300 mg per 24 hours.

The frequency of homocystinuria may be estimated as 1 in 20.000 to 40,000 live births.

Homocystinuris (Fig. 1) is characterized by systemic, ocular and metabolic manifestations.

SYSTEMIC MANIFESTATIONS

The following systemic manifestations are the most important:

Mental retardation

A slowly progressive mental retardation occurs in approximately 50 per cent of the patients. The I.Q. may be very low, ranging from 20-53.

Mental retardation, which may be the result of cerebral vascular disease, is sometimes accompanied by psychomotor retardation. Seizures occur in about 50 per cent of the cases. Spasticity or other neurological signs such as aphasia or muscular paralyses or even schizophrenia have been reported. The EEG may show a diffuse dysrhythmia.

In one series of 3000 mentally defective children, 10 had homocystinuria. The intelligence in homocystinuria may be normal or nearly normal.

Skeletal manifestations

The most charactetistic skeletal abnormality is genu valgum, or knock knees: Fig. 1. Many of the patients typically walk with feet everted in a flat-footed 'Chaplin' or broad-based gait.

Long and thin extremities — arachnodactyly — with a decreases upper segment/lower segment ratio and with joint laxity, as in Marfan's syndrome, are frequent (Fig. 2 and 3). In homocystinuria the dolichostenomelia does

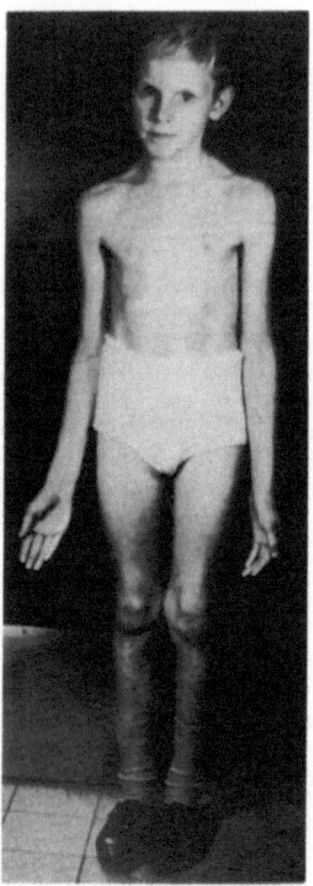

Fig. 1. Homocystinuria, arachnodactyly, genu valgum (pers. obs.).

not exist at birth, but appears later.

Generalized osteoporosis is common. Fractures and destruction of the vertebrae occur with increased frequency. Other skeletal abnormalities are pescavus or flat-foot, pectus excavatum or carinatum, narrowing of the articular spaces, cyphoscoliosis, arched palate, hypoplasia of the mandible, and aplasia of the semilunars.

Anomalies of the skin and hair

The skin is white, fair, dry and covered with red or pink spots, one of which is generally found on the cheek, malar flush. The appearance is manifestly albinoid (Fig. 4). The hair is fair, coarse, sparse and brittle. Livedo reticularis of the trunk and of the extension side of the limbs may be seen.

Abnormal telangiectases around scars and abnormal capillaries in the nail folds have been noted.

The teeth are usually crowded and irregularly aligned.

44

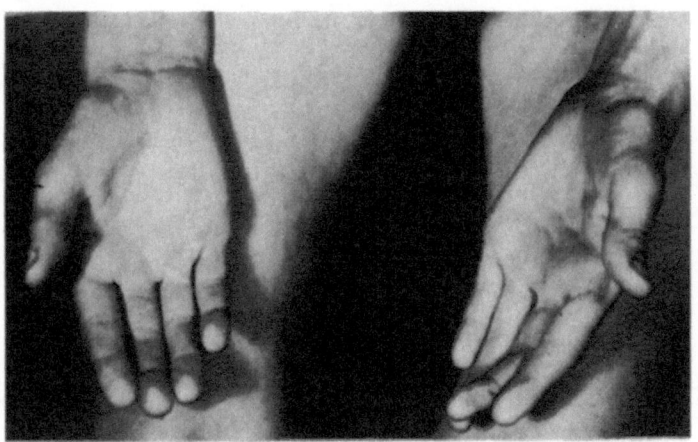

Fig. 2. Homocystinuria, arachnodactyly (pers. obs.).

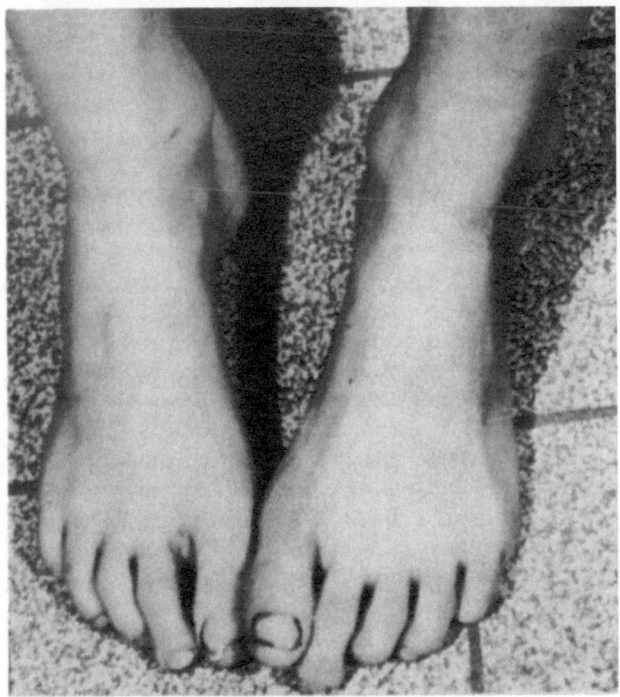

Fig. 3. Homocystinuria, long and slender feet (pers. obs.).

Cardiovascular abnormalities

Thrombo-embolic phenomena in the veins and in the middle-sized arteries is noted in approximately 50 per cent of cases. They are found in the lungs, kidneys, heart and brain. They are more apt to occur after venous or arterial punctures or following general anaesthesia.

Arterial or venous thrombosis explains thrombophlebitis, hypertension,

45

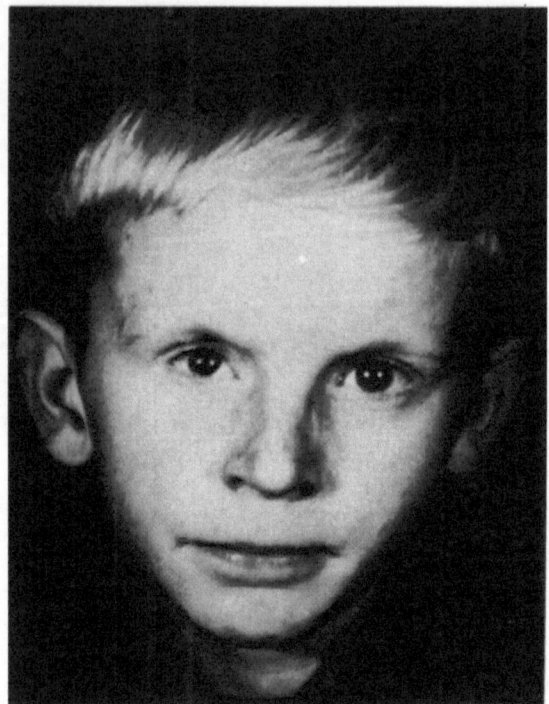
Fig. 4. Homocystinuria, albinoid aspect (pers. obs.).

myocardial infarction, intermittent claudication, acute gangrene of the extremities, cerebro-vascular accidents, gastro-intestinal bleeding due to thrombosis of the mesenteric arteries.

The thrombo-embolic phenomena may be accompanied by blood coagulation disorders or an increased viscosity of the blood due to platelet stickiness. The latter may be related to the homocystine in blood. Moreover, histopathologic examination shows a fibrosis of the intima, together with changes of the elastic fibres and disruption of the media.

The cause of death in patients afflicted with homocystinuria is usually thrombo-embolic phenomena.

Other systemic manifestations are hepatomegaly caused by accumulation of neutral fats in the liver; attacks of respiratory arrest; muscle weakness; chronic pyelonephritis; gluten enteropathy; systemic moniliasis; chronic cor pulmonale and a labile emotional state.

OCULAR MANIFESTATIONS

The most important and constant ocular manifestation is ectopica lentis: Fig. 5. It is seen in at least 90 per cent of cases. There are only a few cases without this manifestation.

The dislocation of the lens generally does not develop before the age of one year, but occurs early in life at a variable age. Downward displacement of the lens is more frequent in homocystinuria than in Marfan's syndrome.

46

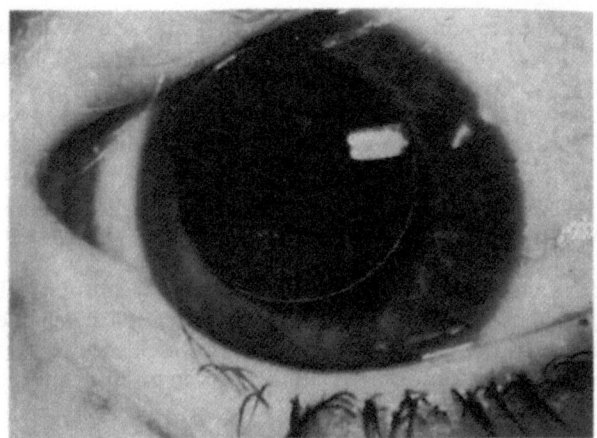

Fig. 5. Homocystinuria, dislocation of the lens (pers. obs.).

The dislocation is progressive and becomes total at 7 years of age or later.

The lens is usually luxated forward, so that pupillary block glaucoma is frequent and often bilateral. This complication may even lead to buphthalmos.

Lens extraction should be avoided for two reasons:

1. General anaesthesia may induce arterial or venous thromboembolism causing the death of the patient.

2. The dangers inherent in the operation itself are great:

a) Vitreous loss is seen in at least 50 per cent of cases

b) Intraocular haemorrhages are frequent.

Hyphema may take several weeks to clear. In a case we saw a vitreous haemorrhage the day after the operation; it cleared after 14 days and then disseminated retinal haemorrhages could be seen. The final result was vision of 0.1. In another case there was already a total hyphema and vitreous haemorrhage the day after surgery. This eye became atrophic.

c) Retinal detachment can also occur.

However, if the visual handicap is too great or if there is a pupillary block glaucoma with high intraocular pressure, operation is mandatory.

The diagnosis of homocystinuria should be considered in all cases of dislocation of the lens even when this appears following trauma.

In exceptional cases homocystinuria may produce clinical signs only in adult age. A homocystinuric patient is known, who became myopic following a slight dislocation of the lens at 43 years of age.

Pathogenesis of the dislocation of the lens

The disorder of homocysteine metabolism may alter collagen, of which cystine is one of the constituents. On the other hand, the zonular fibers, even if they are not collagenous and if they are more similar to elastin, are formed from a protein resistent to collagenase and containing cystine, which is not present in either elastin or collagen, although the amino acid composition is different from that of collagen.

A specific degeneration of the zonular fibers may, however, explain the progressive dislocation of the lens. This was observed with the electron microscope.

Adjacent to the lens the zonular fibers were deficient and recoiled to the surface of the ciliary body, where they lay matted and retracted into a felt work, which fused with a greatly thickened basement membrane of the non-pigmented ciliary epithelium. These changes extended to the pars plana. The non-pigmented epithelium itself showed patchy and pronounced atrophy.

Degenerative changes of the zonular fibers have been found. They were thickened, granular, disorganized and retracted against the thickened basement membrane of the ciliary epithelium with which they were fused. This feltwork was eosinophilic, non fluorescent and non birefringent.

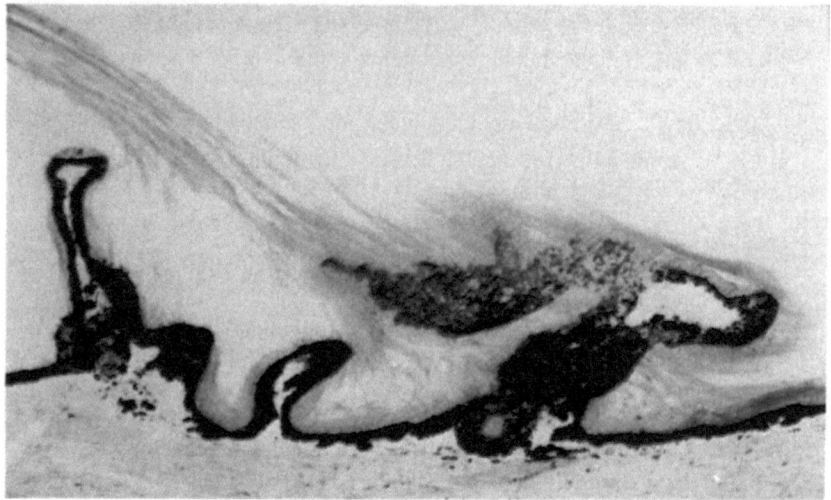

Fig. 6. Homocystinuria (after HENKIND & ASHTON, 1965). Ciliary body with abnormal zonular fibres and intensely stained and thickened basement membrane of the atrophic non-pigmented ciliary epithelium.

Under electron microscopy, thick, PAS positive, amorphous material overlying the non pigmented ciliary epithelium was observed. This material was made up of short segments of zonular fibers, composed of oriented filaments intermingled with short filaments in disarray. The ciliary body itself was atrophic or underdeveloped. The authors could demonstrate that the number of abnormal filament increases with age, while the number of normal zonular fragments decreases with age. Degeneration of the non pigmented ciliary epithelium and of the peripheral neural retina also increases with age.

Hypoplasia of the stroma of ciliary body, the ciliary muscle and ciliary processes, has been described. The non-pigmented ciliary epithelium was covered by a homogeneous, PAS positive material. Lipid deposits were found in the ciliary body and ciliary processes. The stroma of some ciliary processes was hyalinized and contained a homogeneous deposit, composed of small masses with calcified borders.

These observations may be correlated with pigmentations at the retinal periphery and strong adhesions of the vitreous to the ora serrata and pars plana. These were found in spite of a posterior detachment, while the ciliary processes were covered by a grey-whitish membrane.

The dislocation of the lens can be explained by abnormal fibrogenesis of the zonula. This could well result from deprivation of an essential component during development.

Considerable amounts of homocystine and markedly elevated levels of methionine in the aqueous humour of homocystinuric patients with only small traces of cystathionine have been described.

Other ocular manifestations

High myopia of 5 or more diopters occurs in 25 percent of cases. This may be explained by spherophakia.

Light or blue irides are seen in 75 percent of cases and depend on the albinoid appearance. The fundus itself may be albinotic.

Other ocular manifestations are less common. Congenital cataract of the zonular of nuclear type, iris atrophy, diffuse or in patches, optic atrophy apparently unrelated to glaucoma, cystic degeneration of the peripheral retina, retinal detachment, sklerotic changes and sheating of the retinal arteries, uni or bilateral occlusions of the central retinal arteries, retinal dystrophy or chorioretinal atrophy with subnormal electroretinogram and alteration of the photopic response, malformation of the disc with situs inversus, microphthalmos, aniridia, incomplete chorioretinal coloboma, and corectopia have all been reported.

Some ocular findings, such as uveitis, keratitis, hypotony, corneal degeneration, iris atrophy and acquired cataract are probably related to the abnormal anatomic conditions such as dislocated lenses, and not to particular biochemical defects.

Multiple ocular defects may be manifest in 20 per cent of the cases of homocystinuria.

METABOLIC MANIFESTATIONS

Besides paper or column chromatography of the urine, the easiest diagnostic method is the sodium nitroprusside reaction, which readily shows the presence of homocystine. This is known as Brand's rection. Five ml. of urine are mixed with 2 ml. of a 5 per cent solution of sodium cyanide. After 10 minutes, 2 to 4 drops of a 5 per cent solution of sodium nitroprusside are added. If the reaction is positive, the solution immediately becomes bright red, later it fades. The colour is due to reduction of cystine and homocystine to cysteine and homocysteine by the sodium nitroprusside.

Another technique is to place 5 drops of urine and 1 drop of a 10 per cent solution of sodium cyanide in a watch-glass, wait at least 1 minute, and add 1 drop of 1 per cent sodium nitroprusside. The same bright red colour results, if the reaction is positive.

Brand's reaction is not always constant. The automatic analyser for amino acids is more reliable.

The systemic features of homocystinuria with its signs of lens dislocation, mental retardation, albinoid appearance and knock knees is sufficiently characteristic to suggest the diagnosis and to perform a Brand's reaction.
One should realize, however, that there may be no pathologic manifestation.
This should not be surprising since there are also cases of phenylketonuria
without mental retardation and cases of albinism in which pigment is not
absent. In hereditary diseases one may find all degrees of manifestations
from the apparently normal state to the seriously affected one. This variability depends on the interaction between the mutant gene, the normal genes,
and environmental influences.

PROGNOSIS

Patients may die at a young age from occlusive vascular disease. In fact, a
premature death is observed in 40 per cent of cases. Some patients, however, reach the age of 40 years. Mild forms with dislocation of the lens may,
indeed, be seen in adults.

GENETICS

Homocystinuria is transmitted as an autosomal recessive disease, as evidenced by the following:

There are numerous examples of several affected members in one family,
the forbears and descendants being normal.

It would be helpful to be able to recognize the heterozygotes or carriers
of the genes. Until now, this has been possible only in a few cases. It is rare
to find a heterozygote who spontaneously excretes homocystine in the
urine. More commonly, a heterozygote eliminates homocystine, cystine,
after ingestion of an excessive amount of methionine. Liver activity of
cystathionine synthase. More commonly, a heterozygote eliminates homocystine, or cystine, after ingestion affected with homocystinuria. The cystathionine synthase activity can also be estimated in fibroblasts obtained by
tissue culture of the skin.

Phytohemagglutinin stimulated lymphocytes have been used to measure
the cystathionine synthase levels. These are intermediate in heterozygotes,
while they are absent in homozygotes.

DIFFERENTIAL DIAGNOSIS

Homocystinuria must be differentiated from other diseases associated with
dislocation of the lens.

1. Ectopia lentis

Ectopia lentis may be secondary to an exogenous cause such as uveitis,
hypermature cataract or trauma. Its aetiology will then be readily recognized.

If ectopia lentis is heredo-familial, the following variations may occur:

50

1. It may be isolated and transmitted as an autosomal dominant trait.
2. It may be associated with ectopia of the pupil and transmitted as an autosomal recessive trait. The ectopia of the pupil and the absence of other abnormalities allow identification of this entity.
3. Besides homocystinuria, a dislocation of the lens may be seen in Marchesani's syndrome and in Marfan's syndrome; two examples of hereditary dystrophy of the connective tissue.

2. Marfan's syndrome

The ocular and skeletal disorders of homocystinuria may cause it to be mistaken for Marfan's syndrome (Fig. 7 and 8). Patients with homocys-

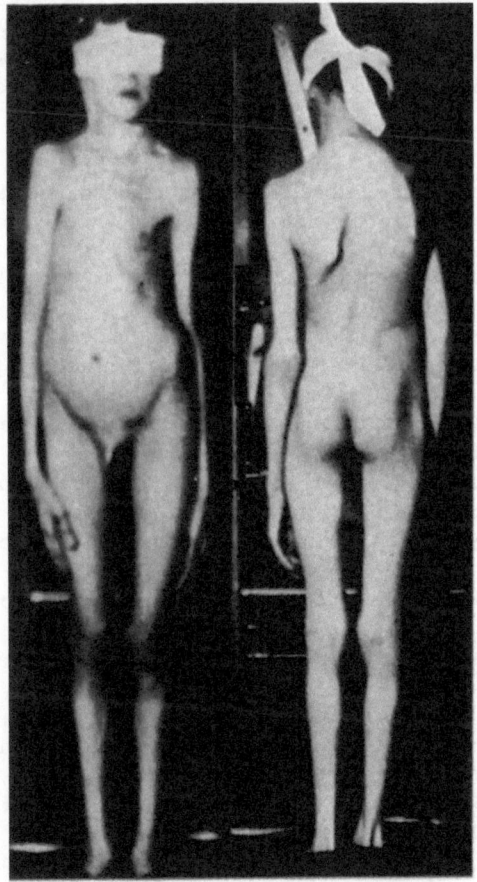

Fig. 7. Marfan's syndrome (pers. obs.).

tinuria have, indeed, been reported as having Marfan's disease. In the presence of a Marfan's syndrome, Brand reaction should be included.

The most important differences between homocystinuria and Marfan's

51

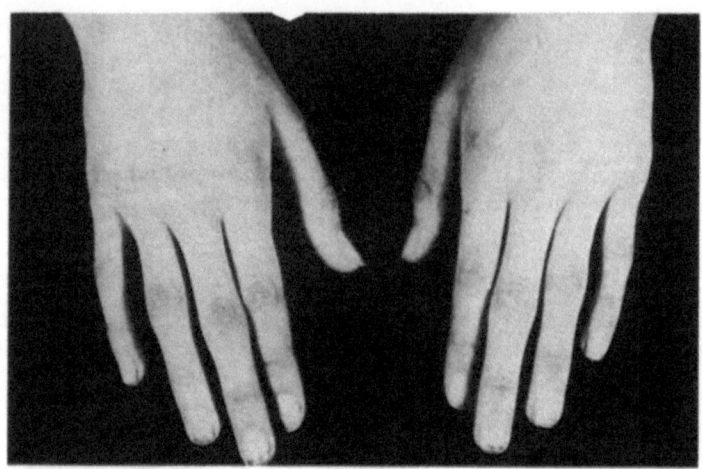

Fig. 8. Arachnodactyly in Marfan's syndrome (pers. obs.).

syndrome are (Table I):
1. In Marfan's disease the dislocation of the lens, which exist in at least 80 per cent of cases, is mostly upwards and inwards, while in homocystinuria it is mostly downwards.

It is worthwhile to mention that in Marchesani's syndrome the dislocation of the lens is mostly upwards and outwards.
2. In Marfan's disease the dislocation of the lens is nearly always partial and nearly always not progressive, while in homocystinuria it is progressive and becomes complete after seven years of age.
3. In Marfan's disease a peripapillary choroidal sclerosis is frequent, while in homocystinuria the fundus is usually normal.
4. In Marfan's disease the typical arachnodactyly is already present at birth. It should be confirmed by radiological determination of the metacarpal index. In homocystinuria arachnodactyly is not present at birth, but develops later.
5. In Marfan's disease, there is no osteoporosis. In homocystinuria it is nearly constant.
6. In Marfan's disease there is no genu valgum. It is also nearly constant in homocystinuria.
7. In Marfan's disease, there may be a cardiopathy and even aortic aneurism, but no thromboembolic phenomena, while in homocystinuria there is no cardiopathy, but arterial and venous thromboses.
8. In Marfan's disease there is no albinoid aspect with malar flush, which is regularly seen in homocystinuria.
9. In Marfan's disease, there is no mental retardation, which is frequently seen in homocystinuria.
10. In Marfan's disease hydroxyproline is found in the urine, but no homocystine, while in homocystinuria no hydroxyproline is found.

The urinary hydroxyproline excretion is increased in the urine of Marfan's patients while the hydroxyproline level is decreased in the serum.
11. Marfan's disease is autosomal dominant with variable expressivity while

52

TABLE I

	Dislocation of the lens	Other ocular abnormalities	Skeletal abnormalities	Cardio-vascular abnormalities	Cutaneous abnormalities	Mental retardation	Urine	Genetics
Homocystinuria	acquired, nearly constant after 1 year, downwards, progressive, complete after 7 years	myopia spherophakia	arachnodactyly, but not present at birth, genu valgum osteoporosis	arterial and venous thrombosis, no cardiopathy	albinoid aspect, red spots on skin, malar flush, livedo reticularis	frequent	homocystine	autosomal recessive
Marfan's syndrome	congenital, nearly constant, upwards, partial, rarely progressive	peripapillary choroidal sclerosis	congenital arachnodactyly, no osteoporosis	cardiopathy no vascular thrombosis	no cutaneous changes	absent	hydroxyproline, Brand's reaction negative	autosomal dominant dominant
Marchesani's	frequent, as in Marfran's syndrome	micro- and spherophakia	Brachymorphy	absent	no cutaneous changes	absent	no abnormal amino acids	autosomal dominant or recessive

53

homocystinuria is an autosomal recessive disease.

TREATMENT

Theoretically, a diet low methionine and high in cystine should be able to arrest the progress of the disease, at least in those cases that have been detected early. The efficacy of such a diet has been confirmed. Perhaps supplementary cystathionine may be necessary. On the other hand, dietary restriction, in addition to the failure to completely normalize the biochemical abnormalities, may have a damaging effect by the diet itself. Oral folic acid therapy in two patients brought about a decrease in the urinary excretion of homocystine and an increase in methionine excretion.

Pyridoxine, also known as vitamin B_6, stimulates one or other pathway of methionine or homocysteine metabolism (250 to 500 mg daily). Several homocystinuric patients were treated in this manner. Five hundred mg of vitamin B_6 daily brought the amino acids of the urine, plasma, and red blood cells of two siblings back to normal. A third patient responded transiently, but later became resistant to the beneficial effect of 1500 mg pyridoxine daily, whereas her cousin, possibly heterozygous and much less severely afflicted, was controlled by 50 mg pyridoxine daily. Platelet stickiness, which is related to the concentration of homocystine in the blood, was partially corrected by the treatment in all four cases. Hair texture and colour returned to normal in one case.

Pyridoxine treatment has afterwards been tried with variable results. Pyridoxine treatment will complement, but not supplement, a less strictly methionine-poor and cystine-rich diet. We know a case, without ectopia of the lens, which was biochemically completely normalized by pyridoxine and a diet poor in methionine and rich in cystine. So far it is impossible to say if this treatment, pyridoxinw and diet, can prevent or halt dislocation of the lens.

As pyridoxine was successfully used in one patient out of three, some authorities believe that there are two types of homocystinuria, one being vitamin B_6 dependent and the other not. At the present two types of homocystinuria are accepted: a vitamin B_6-sensitive and a non-vitamin B_6 sensitive form.

CONCLUSION

When a child has ectopia of the lens, one must always consider the possibility of homocystinuria, a diagnosis that can be made with reasonable certainty by the detection of other clinical manifestations such as mental retardation, skeletal abnormalities, genu valgum and arrachnodactyly, and albinoid features, skin dotted with red spots, malar flush and blond hair. A simple test of the urine, the sodium nitroprusside reaction, can confirm the diagnosis.

REFERENCES

APPELMANS M., MISSOTTEN L., KEMP M. & REITER M. Homocystinurie. *Bull. Soc. Belge Ophtal.*, 156: *638-650* (1970).

ARNOTTE E.J. & GREAVES D.P. Ocular involvement in homocystinuria. *Brit. J. Ophthal.* 48: *688-689 (1964)*.

BARBER G.W. & SPAETH G.L. Pyridoxine therapy in homocystinuria. *Lancet,* 1: *337* (1967).

BESSIERE E., VERIN P. & LE REBELLER M.J. − Biopsies cutanées et recherches d'acides aminés urinaires dans les ectopies cristalliniennes. *Bull. Soc. Ophtal. France* 67: *1028-1031* (1967).

BONAMOUR G. & POMMIER M.L. Luxation du cristallin et homocystinurie. *Ophtalmologica (Basel),* 156: *267,* 1968.

BRANCATO R. & COTROZZI G. L'omocistinuria. Rivista sintetica. *Ann. Ottal.,* 94: *996-1010* (1968).

BRENTON D.P. & CUSWORTH D.C. Homocystinuria: metabolism of (35 S) methionine. *Clin Sci.,* 31: *197* (1966).

BRENTON D.P., CUSWORTH D.C., DENT C.E. & JONES E.E. Homocystinuria: clinical and dietary studies. *Quart. J. Med.,* 35: *325* (1966).

BRENTON D.P., CUSWORTH D.C. & GAULL G.E. Homocystinuria; biochemcial studies of tissues, including a comparison with cysthathioninuria. *Pediatrics,* 35: *50* (1965a).

BRENTON D.P., CUSWORTH D.C. & GAULL G.E. Homocystinuria; metabolic studies on 3 patients. *J. Pediat.,* 67: *58-68* (1965b).

BRETT E.M. Homocystinuria with epilepsy. *Proc. roy. Soc. Med.,* 59: *484* (1966).

CAREY M.C., DONOVAN D.E., FITZGERALD O. & MCAULEY F.D. Homocystinuria. *Amer. J. Med.,* 45: *7* (1968a).

CAREY M., FENNELLY J.J. & FITZGERALD O. Folate metabolism in homocystinuria. *Irish J. Med. Sci.,* 6: *488* (1966).

CAREY M.C., FENNELLY J.J. & FITZGERALD O. Homocystinuria. *Amer. J. Med.,* 45: *26* (1968).

CARSON N.A.J. Homocystinuria; trial treatment of a 5-year-old severely retarded child with a natural diet low in methionine. *J. Dis. Child.,* 113: *95* (1967).

CARSON N.A.J. Homocystinuria. *Proc. Roy. Soc. Med.,* 63: *41-43* (1970).

CARSON N.A.J. & CARRE I.J. Treatment of homocystinuria with pyridoxine. *Arch. Dis. Child.,* 44: *387,* 1969.

CARSON N.A.J., CUSWORTH D.C., DENT C.E., FIELD C.M.B., NEILL D.W. & WESTWALL R.D. Homocystinuria, a new inborn error of metabolism associated with mental deficiency. *Arch. Dis. Childh.,* 38: *425* (1963).

CARSON N.A.J., DENT C.E., FIELD C.M.B. & GAULL G.E. Homocystinuria; clinical and pathological review of 10 cases. *J. Pediat.,* 66: *565-583,* (1965).

CARSON N.A.J. & NEILL D.W. Metabolic abnormalities detected in a survey of mentally backward individuals in Northern Ireland. *Arch. Dis. Childh.,* 37: *505,* (1962).

CERENEA P. & LUPESCU E. Homocystinuria and arachnodactyly. *Ophthalmologia, Bucarest,* 15: *99-106* (1971).

CHASE H.P., GOODMANS S.I. & O'BRIEN D. Treatment of homocystinuria. *Arch. Dis. Childh.,* 42: *514* (1967).

CHOU S.M. & WAISMAN H.A. Spongy degeneration of the central nervous system; case of homocystinuria. *Arch. Path.,* 79: *357* (1965).

CLINE J.W., GOYER R.A., LIPTON J. & MASON R.G. Adult homocystinuria with ectopia lentis. *8th Med. J. (Bgham),* 64: *613-617* (1971).

COGAN D.G. Ocular correlates of inborn metabolic defects. *Canad. med. Ass. J.,* 95: *1055* (1966).

CROSS H.E. & JENSEN A.D. Ocular manifestations in the Marfan syndrome and homocystinuria. *Amer. J. Ophtal.,* 75: *405-420* (1973).

CURTUIS H.C., MARTENET A.C. & ANDERS P.W. Bestimmung von freien Aminosäuren im Augenkammerwasser des Menschen bei Homocystinuriepatienten und Kontrolfallen. *Clin. Chim. Acta,* 19: *469* (1968).

DANIS P., HUBERT J.M. & MASSIEN V. Homocystinurie. Étude histologique oculaire. *Bull. Soc. Belge Ophtal.,* 162: *850-857* (1972).

DAYRAS J.C., SOURDILLE J., DELTHIL P. & LECLERCQ C. A propos d'un cas d'homocystinurie. *Gaz. Méd. France,* 77: *103-111* (1970).

55

DECKERS P.F.L. Biochemische afwijkingen bij het syndroom van Marfan. *Ned. Tijdschr. Geneesk.*, 116: *737-740* (1972).
DEXTER M.W., LAWTON A.H. & WARREN L.O. Marfan's syndrome with aortic thrombosis. *Arch. Intern. Med.*, 99: *485* (1957).
DUNN H.G., PERRY T.L. & DOLMAN C.L. Homocystinuria: a recently discovered cause of mental defect and cerebro-vascular thrombosis. *Neurology (Minneap.)*, 16: *407* (1966).
DUTHIE O.M. Discussion of the paper of P. HENKIND & N. ASHTON. *Trans Ophthal. Soc. U.K.*, 85: *37-38* (1965).
EDITORIAL. Dislocated lenses and homocystinuria. *Arch. Ophtal.*, 74: *446-447* (1965).
FALLS H.F. Discussion of the communication of G.L. Spaeth and G.W. Barber, Homocystinuria. *Trans. Amer. Acad. Ophthal. Otolaryng.*, 69: *829-830* (1965).
FEUVRIER Y.M., BOIXEL J. & DONNIOU G. Homocystinurie. Une observation. *Bull. Soc. Ophtal. France*, 68: *280-284* (1968).
FIELD C.M.B., CARSON N.A.J., CUSWORTH D.C., DENT C.E. & NEILL D.W. Homocystinuria; a new disorder of metabolism. Abstract from the X International Congress of Pediatrics, Lisboa, p. 274, (1962).
FINKELSTEIN J.D., MUDD S.H., IRREVERRE F. & LASTER L. Homocystinuria due to cystathionine synthetase deficiency; the mode of inheritance. *Science*, 146: *785* (1964).
FRANÇOIS J. Manifestations oculaires dans certaines erreurs congénitales du métabolisme. *Ann. méd. Nancy*, 6: *253-271* (1967).
FRANÇOIS J. Manifestations oculaires dans l'homocystinurie et la glycolipidose de Fabry. *Bull. Soc. Ophtal. Fr.*, 67: *1001-1017* (1968a).
FRANÇOIS J. Ocular manifestations in certain congenital errors of metabolism. In: Congenital anomalies of the eye, pp. 157-198, Mosby, Saint Louis, (1968b).
FRANÇOIS J. Homocystinuria. In: *Perspectives in Ophthalmology*, II, Excerpta Medica, Monograph, *81-95*, (1970).
FRANÇOIS J. Ocular manifestations in aminoacidopathies. Monographs in Human Genetics, S. Karger, Basel, 6: *99-113* (1972).
FRANÇOIS J. Ocular manifestations in amino-acidopathies. *Adv. Ophthal.*, S. Karger, Basel, 25: *28-103* (1972).
FRANÇOIS J. & COPPIETERS R. Homocystinurie. *Bull. Soc. Belge Ophtal.*, 147: *485-494* (1967).
FRANÇOIS J., GAUDIER B., ASSEMAN R., SINGER J.C. & NUYTS J.P. L'homocystinurie. *Bull. Soc. Ophtal. France*, 67: *827-830* (1967).
FRANÇOIS P., GAUDIER B., PRUYOT J. & SINGER J.C. La rétine dans l'homocystinurie. *Bull. Soc. Ophtal. France*, 68: *562-564* (1967).
FREYCON F. & FREYCONN M.T. L'homocystinurie. *Pédiatrie*, 20: *495* (1965).
FREZZOTTI R., BARDELLI A.M., FOIS A. & TESTAFERRATA A. Presentazione di casi di omocistinuria con alterazioni oculari. *Boll. Oculistica*, 50: *91-113* (1971).
GARSTON J.B., GORDON R.R., HART C.T. & POLLITT R.J. An unusual case of homocystinuria. *Brit. J. Ophthal.*, 54: *248-251*, (1970).
GAUDIER B., FRANÇOIS P., BISERTE G., NUYTS J.P. & BOMBART E. L'homocystinurie. *Pédiatrie*, 21: *889* (1966).
GAUDIER B., FRANÇOIS P., BISERTE G., DAUTREVAUX M., NUYTS J.P. & BOMBART E. L'homocystinurie. *Arch. franç. Pédiat.*, 25: *541*, (1968).
GAULL G.E. The pathogenesis of homocystinuria; implications for treatment. *J. Dis. Child.*, 113: *103* (1967).
GAULL G.E., CUSWORTH D.C., BRENTON D.P. & DENT G.E. The biochemical defect in homocystinuria. *J. Pediat.*, 65: *1409* (1964).
GAULL G.E. & GAITONDE M.K. Homocystinuria; an observation on the inheritance of cystathionine synthase deficiency. *J. med. Genet.*, 3: *194-197* (1966).
GAULL G.E., RASSIN D.K. & STURMAN J.A. Pyridoxine dependency in homocystinuria. *Lancet*, 2: *1302* (1968).
GERRITSEN T. The unusual finding of homocystine excretion in an infant. *Fed. Proc.*, 22: *650* (1963).
GERRITSEN T., VAUGHAN J.G. & WAISMAN H.A. The identification of

homocystine in the urine. *Biochem. biophys. Res. Commun.*, 9: *493* (1962).
GERRITSEN T. & WAISMAN H.A. Homocystinuria; absence of cystathionine in the brain. *Science*, 145: *588* (1964a).
GERRITSEN T. & WAISMAN H.A. Homocystinuria, an error in the metabolism of methionine. *Pediatrics.*, 33: *413-420*, 1964b.
GERRITSEN T. & WAISMAN H.A. Homocystinuria. In: J.B. Stanbury et al. (Ed.). The metbolic basis of inherited disease, 2nd ed., p. 420, Mc Graw-Hill, New York (1966).
GERRITSEN T. & WAISMAN H.A. Homocystinuria. Cystathionine synthase deficiency. In: J.B. Stanbury, J.B. Wijngaarden and D.S. Frederickson: The metabolic basis of inherited disease, Mc Graw-Hill, New York, 404-412: (1972).
GFELLER J. & BUDLIGER H. Homocystinuria and os lunatum. *Lancet*, 2: *548* (1966).
GIBSON J.B., CARSON N.A.J. & NIELL D.W. Pathological findings in homocystinuria. *J. Clin. Path.*, 17: *427-437* (1964).
GIRARD P.F., SCHOTT B., BADY B., BOUCHER M. & DAVID M. Observation d'homocystinurie familiale avec altérations carotidiennes et luxation du cristallin. *Lyon méd.*, 218: *1369* (1967).
GOLDSTEIN J.L., CAMPBELL B.K. & GARTLER S.M. Homocystinuria. Heterozygote-detection using phytohemagglutinin stimulated lymphocytes. *J. Clin. Invest.*, 52: *218-221* (1973).
GOUX J.P. & KALLAY O. Les complications oculaires des erreurs congénitales du métabolisme. *Bull. Soc. Belge Ophtal.*, 157: *10-319*, (1971).
GREER W. & WILLIAMS C.M. Diagnosis of homocystinuria by gas-chromatography. *Analyt. Biochem.*, 19: *40* (1967).
GUIHARD J., FELLOUSE J.C., LANIECE M. & SIGNORET C. Une erreur innée du métabolisme. L'homocystinurie. *J. Méd. Caen*, 7: *5-13* (1972).
GUPTE S.D., JAIN I.S. & KUMAR J. Acquired cataract in homocystinuria. *Indian J. Ophthal.*, 19: *49-51* (1971).
HALL W.K., CORYELL M.E., HOLLOWELL J.G. Jr. & THEVAOS T.G. A metabolic study of homocystinuria. *Fed. Proc.*, 24: *470* (1965).
HAMBRAEUS L., WRANNE L. & LORENTSSON R. Biochemical and therapeutic studies in two cases of homocystinuria. *Clin. Sci.*, 35: *457* (1968).
HARNAGEA E., BARBULESCU G., BOTEZ O. & STURDZA R. Clinical and genetic aspects in Marfan's syndrome. *Oftalmologia, Bucarest*, 14: *351-356* (1970).
HEILMANN K., SUSCHKE J. & MURKEN J.D. Marfansyndrom. Ophthalmologische, klinische, biochemische und genetische Untersuchungen. *Ber. Dtsche Ophthal. Ges.*, 70: *457-461* (1969).
HENKIND P. & ASHTON N. Homocystinuria. *Brit. Med. J.*, 5371: *1485* (1963).
HENKIND P. & ASHTON N. Ocular pathology in homocystinuria. *Trans. Ophthal. Soc. U.K.*, 85: *21-37* (1965).
HINDLE N.W. & CRAWFORD J.S. Dislocation of the lens in Marfan's syndrome. Its effect and treatment. *Canad. J. Ophthal.*, 4: *128-135* (1969).
HOOFT C., CARTON D. & SAMIJN W. Pyridoxine treatment in homocystinuria. *Lancet*, 1: *1384* (1967).
HOPE D.B. Cystathionine accumulation in brains of pyridoxine deficient rats. *J. Neurochem.*, 11: *327* (1964).
JAROSZEWICS A. & KOSSOWICZ H. Ocular involvement in homocystinuria. *Klin. Oczna*, 41: *853-857* (1971).
JENSEN A.D. & CROSS H.E. Surgical treatment of dislocated lenses in the Marfan syndrome and homocystinuria. *Trans. Amer. Acad. Ophthal.*, 76: *1491-1499* (1972).
JOHNSTON S.S. Pupil-block glaucoma in homocystinuria. *Brit. J. Ophthal.*, 52: *251-256* (1968).
KENNEDY C., SHIV V.E. & ROWLAND L.P. Homocystinuria: a report in two siblings. *Pediatrics*, 36: *736* (1965).
KLAVINDS J.V. Pathology of amino acid excess. I. Effects of administration of excessive amounts of sulphur containing amino acids; homocystinuria. *Brit. J. Exp. Path.*, 44: *507* (1963).
KOMROWER G.M., LAMBERT A.M., CUSWORTH D.C. & WESTALL R.G. Dietary

treatment of homocystinuria. *Arch. dis. Childh.*, 41: *466-671* (1966).
KOMROWER G.M., LAMBERT A.M., CUSWORTH D.C. & WESTALL R.G. Dietary treatment of homocystinuria. *J. Dis. Child.*, 113: *98* (1967).
KOMROWER G.M. & WILSON V.K. Homocystinuria. *Proc. roy. Soc. Med.*, 56: *993-997* (1963).
LARMANDE A. & JEZEGABEL C. Le syndrome de Marchesani. Étude critique et acquisitions récentes. *Ann. Oculistique, Paris*, 204: *819-832* (1971).
LASTER L., MUDD S.H., FINKELSTEIN J.D. & IRREVERRE F. Homocystinuria due to cystathionine synthetase deficiency; the metabolism of Methionine. *J. Clin. Invest.*, 44: *1708* (1965).
LASTER L., SPAETH G.L., MUDD S.H. & FINKELSTEIN J.D. Homocystinuria due to cytathionine synthetase deficiency. *Ann. intern. Med.*, 63: *1117* (1965).
LE CLERCQ C. L'homocystinurie. *Arch. Méd. Normandie*, 7: *527-532* (1972).
LIEBERMANN T.W., PODIS S.M. & HARTSTEIN H. Acute glaucoma, ectopia lentis and homocystinuria. *Amer. J. Ophthal.*, 61: *252-255* (1966).
LOUGHRIDGE L.W. Renal abnormalities in the Marfan syndrome. *Quart. J. Med.*, 28: *531* (1959).
LYNAS M.A. Marfan's syndrome in Northern Ireland, an account of 13 families. *Ann. hum. Genet.*, 22: *289* (1958).
MARTENET A.C., CURTIS H.C. & ANDERS P.W. Altérations oculaires de l'homocystinure. 2. Les acides aminés de l'humeur aqueuse. *Arch. Ophtal. (Paris)*, 28: *295-302, Ophthalmologica (Basel)*, 156: *262* (1967).
MARTENET A.C., WITMER R. & SPEISER P. Altérations oculaires dans l'homocystinurie. *Ophthalmologica*, 154: *318-323* (1967).
MATSUMOTO K. & HAMAI Y. Cystinosis and homocystinuria. Report of a case. *Rinsho Ganka*, 24: *839-845* (1970).
MCDONALD L., BRAY C., FIELD C., LOVE F. & DAVIS B. Homocystinuria, thrombosis and the blood platelets, *Lancet*, 1: *745* (1964).
MCKUSICK V.A., HALL J.G. & CHAR F. The clinical and genetic characteristics of homocystinuria. In: Inherited disorders of Sulphur metabolism. Proc. VIII Symp. Soc. Study of Inborn Errors of Metabolism, Belfast, 1970, Edited by N.A.J. Carson and D.N. Raine, Livingstone, London, (1971).
MUDD S.H. Homocystinuria. The known cases. In: Inherited disorders of Sulphur Metabolism. Proc. VIII Symp. Soc. Study of Inborn Errors of Metabolism, Belfast, 1970, edited by N.A.J. Carson and D.N. Raine, Livingstone, London (1971).
MUDD S.H., FINKELSTEIN J.D., IRREVERRE F. & LASTER L. Homocystinuria; an enzymatic defect. *Science*, 143: *1443*, (1964).
MUDD S.H., FINKELSTEIN J.D., IRREVERRE R. & LASTER L. Threonine dehydrates activity in humans lacking cystathionine synthetase. *Biochem.\biophys. Res. Commun.*, 19: *665* (1965).
MUKUNO K., MATSUI K. & HARAGUCHI H. Ocular manifestations of homocystinuria; report of two cases. *Acta Soc. Ophthal. Jap.*, 71: *66-73* (1967).
PERRY T.L., DUNN H.G., HANSEN S., MCDOUGALL L. & WARRINGTON P.D. Early diagnosis and treatment of homocystinuria. *Pediatrics*, 37: *503-505*, (1966a).
PERRY T.L., HANSEN S., BAR H.P. & MCDOUGALL L. Homocystinuria; excretion of a new sulfur-containing amino acid in urine. *Science*, 152: *776* (1966b).
PERRY T.L., HANSEN S. & MCDOUGALL L. Homolanthionine. excretion homocystinuria. *Science*, 152: *1750* (1966c).
PERRY T.L., HANSEN S., MCDOUGALL L. & WARRINGTON P.D. Sulfur-containing amino-acids in the plasma and urine of homocystinuria. *Clin. Chim. Acta*, 15: *409* (1967).
PETRYKOWSKI V. Zur Frühdiagnose und Pathogenese der Homocystinurie. *Dtsche med. Wschr.*, 93: *1877* (1968).
PIETRUSCHKA G. & PRIESS G. Zur klinischen Symptomatik und Prognose des Marfan und Marchesani Syndroms. *Klin. Mbl. Augenheilk.*, 159: *468-478* (1971).
PRESLEY G.D. & SIDBURY J.B. Homocystinuria and ocular defects. *Amer. J. Ophthal.*, 63: *1723-1727* (1967).
PRESLEY G.D., STINSON I.N. & SIDBURY J.B. Homocystinuria at the North Carolina State School for the Blind. *Amer. J. Ophthal.*, 66: *884-889* (1968).
PRESLEY G.D., STINSON I.N. & SIDBURY J.B. Ocular defects associated with

homocystinuria. Sth Med. J. (bgham), 62: *944-946* (1969).

PRICE J., VICKERS C.F.H. & BROOKER B.K. A case of homocystinuria with noteworthy dermatological features. *J. Ment. Defic. Res.*, 12: *111* (1968).

QUERE M.A., ROSSAZZA C. & DELPLACE M.D. A propos d'un cas d'homocystinurie. *Bull. Soc. Ophtal. France*, 71: *388-391* (1971).

RAHMAN M. Homocystinuria. Review of four cases. *Brit. J. Ophthal.*, 55: *338-342* (1971).

RAMSEY M.S., YANOFF M. & FINE B.S. The ocular histopathology of homocystinuria. A light and electron microscopic study. *Amer. J. Ophthal.*, 74: *377-385* (1972).

SALADO F. & VALLS A. Homocistinuria. *Arch. Soc. Esp. Oftal.*, 31: *365-376* (1971).

SALOMONS G., KELESKE L. & OPITZ E. Evaluation of the effects of terminating the diet in phenulketonuria. *J. Pediat.*, 69: *596* (1966).

SANCHEZ R.B. & CABALLERO M.L.R. Subluxation of the lens, microspherophakia and homocystinuria. *Arch. Soc. Esp. Oftal.*, 31: *545-568* (1971).

SARDHARWALLA I.B., JACKSON S.H., HAWKE H.D. & SASS KORTSAK A. Homocystinuria, a study with low methionine diet in three patients. *Canad. med. Ass. J.*, 99: *731* (1968).

SCHIMKE R.N., MCKUSICK V.A., HUANG T. & POLLACK A.D. Homocystinuria studies of 20 families with 38 affected members. *J. Amer. med. Ass.*, 193: *711-719* (1965a).

SCHIMKE R.N., MCKUSICK V.A., & POLLACK A.D. Homocystinuria simulating Marfan's syndrome. *Trans. Ass. Amer. Phycns*, 78: *60* (1965b).

SCHIMKE R.M., MCKUSICK V.A. & WEILBAECHER R.G. Homocystinuria. In: Amino Acid Metabolism and Genetic Variation (W.L. Nyhan), Mc Graw-Hill, New York (1967).

SCHNEIDER A.J. & GARRARD S.D. Diagnostic and therapeutic implications of persistent hyperphenylalaninemia in an infant heterozygous for the gene of phenylketonuria. *J. Pediat.*, 68: *704* (1966).

SENSENBRENNER J.A. Homocystinuria with vascular complications. Birth defects. *Orig. Art. Ser.*, 8: *286-287* (1972).

SHIPMAN R.T. Homocystinuria. Some old clinical presentations and some pitfalls in diagnosis. *Aust. J. Ment. Retard.*, 1: *94-96* (1970).

SOURDILLE J., DELTHIL P., LEGRAS M. & DAYRAS J. L'homocystinurie, cause possible de cécité de l'enfant. *Bull. Soc. Franç. Ophtal.*, 82: *16-21* (1969).

SOURDILLE J. & LEGRAS M. L'homocystinurie. Ses pièges. Bull. Soc. Belge Ophthal., 157 *350-353* (1971).

SPAETH G.L. Homocystinuria; the significance of its successful treatment. *Trans. Ophthal. Soc. U.K.*, 88: *47-78* (1968).

SPAETH G.L. & BARBER G.W. Homocystinuria in a mentally retarded child and her normal cousin. *Trans. Amer. Acad. Ophthal. Otolaryng.*, 69: *912-930* (1965).

SPAETH G.L. & BARBER G.W. Homocystinuria: its ocular manifestations. *J. Pediat. Ophthal.*, 3: *42-48* (1966).

SPAETH G.L. & BARBER G.W. Prevalence of homocystinuria among the mentally retarded; evaluation of a specific screening test. *Pediatrics*, 40: *586* (1967).

SPIRO H.R., SCHIMKE R.N. & WELSH J.P. Schizophrenia in a patient with a defect in methionine metabolism. *J. Nerv. ment. Dis.*, 141: *285* (1965).

STRAATSMA B.R., ALLEN R.A., PETIT T.H. & HALL M.O. Subluxation of the lens treated with iris photocoagulation. *Amer. J. Ophthal.*, 61: *1312-1324* (1966).

SZABO G. & BOLCS S. The homocystinuric syndrome. *Szemészet*, 106: *155-158* (1969).

TADA K., YOSHIDA T., HIRONO H. & ARAKAWA T. Homocystinuria: amino-acid pattern of the liver. *Tohoku J. exp. Med.*, 92: *325* (1967).

TANCREDI F., FIORE C., DE PAOLA E. & AURICCHIO S. Su di un caso di omocistinuria. *Minerva pediat.*, 19: *642* (1967).

THOMAS R.P., HOLLOWELL J.G., PETERS H.J., CORYELL M.E. & LASTER R.H. Homocystinuria and ectopia lentis in Negro family. *J. Amer. med. Ass.*, 198: *560-562* (1966).

TURNER B. Pyridoxine treatment in homocystinuria. *Lancet*, 2: *1151* (1967).

TURNER G., DEY J. & TURNER B. Homocystinuria; a report of two Australian families. *Aust. paediat. J.,* 3: *48* (1967).
VARGA B. & MCKUSICK V.A. On the relationship between homocystinuria and Marfan-syndrome. *Orv. Hetil.,* 108: *969* (1967).
WAISMAN H.A. & GERRITSEN T. Homocystinuria; an error in the metabolism of methionine. *Pediatrics,* 33: *413* (1964).
WAISMAN H.A., GERRITSEN T., VAUGHAN J.G. & KAVEGGIA E. Methioninemia and homocystinuria, a new error of metabolism. Abstract from the 73rd Annual Meeting of the American Pediatrics Society, p. 51 (1963).
WAKUSAWA S., TAKAKU I., SATO Y., KIMURA R. & YOSHIDA T. Ocular involvement in homocystinuria. *Rinsho Ganka,* 23: *869-874* (1969).
WELCH J.P., CLOWER C.G. & SCHIMKE R.N. The pink spot in schizophrenics and its absence in homocystinurics. *Brit. J. Psychiat.,* 115: *163* (1969).
WERDER E.A., CURTIS H.C., TANCREDI F., ANDERS P.W. & PRADER A. Homocystinurie. *Helv. paediat. Acta,* 21: *1* (1966).
WHITE H.A., ARAKI S., THOMPSON H.L., BOWLAND L.P. & COWEN D. Homocystinuria. *Trans. Amer. Neurol. Ass.,* 89: *24* (1964).
WHITE H.K., ROWLAND P., ARAKI S., THOMPSON H.L. & COWEN D. Homocystinuria. *Arch. Neurol. (Chic.),* 13: *455* (1965).
WILSON R.S. & RUIZ R.S. Bilateral central retinal artery occlusion in homocystinuria. A case report. *Arch. Ophthal., Chicago,* 82: *267-268* (1969).
WOLLENSAK J. Homocystinurie und Linsenektopie. *Graefes Arch. Ophthal.,* 169: *357* (1966).
WOLLENSAK J. Syndroma Marfan und Homocystinurie. *Ber. dtsch. ophthal. Ges.,* 68: *404-407* (1967).
WOLLENSAK J. Das Auge und die angeborenen Stoffwechselstörungen des Bindesgewebes. *Klin. Mbl. Augenheilk.,* 154: *473* (1969).
WRIGHT L.D. An inborn error of metabolism associated with deficiency of enzyme cystathionine synthetase leading to homocystinuria. *New York St. J. Med.,* 65: *559* (1965).
YAMORI K. Studies on free amino-acids in the urine of patients with ocular disease. Report II: hydroxyproline in the urine of patients with Marfan's syndrome. *Folia Ophthal. Jap.,* 20: *600-606* (1969).
YOSHIDA T., TADA K., YOKOYAMA Y. & ARAKAWA P. Homocystinuria of Vitamin B_6 dependent type. *Tohoku J. exp. Med.,* 96: *235* (1968).

KATAMNESTIC EXAMINATIONS AND GENETIC INVESTIGATIONS ON MARRIAGES, CHILDREN AND SOCIAL STATUS OF 196 BLIND FORMER PUPILS OF A SCHOOL FOR THE BLIND

W. JAEGER & A. BLANKENAGEL

(Heidelberg, West Germany)

Prevention of blindness activities in the future will be increasingly concerned with persons afflicted with hereditary forms of blindness.

For almost 100 years the Hospital for Ophthalmology of the University of Heidelberg supervised the Ilvesheim School for the Blind. Complete medical reports and bulletins of young patients are available; these records having survived destruction during the Second World War.

Statistics from this school compiled previously showed that the causes of blindness have radically changed. At the end of the 19th Century 30% of all pupils at this school had lost their vision as a result of disease of the cornea, such as postblenorrheic leucomas. This cause of blindness has now virtually disappeared; on the other hand, hereditary, gene-determined forms of blindness are increasing.

In view of this for the past ten years, in conjunction with our colleagues of the Institute for Human Genetics, we have providing genetic counseling to pupils who left this school of the blind. In order to be on firm ground, we have carried out katamnestic investigations on all accessible ex-pupils of the Ilvesheim School. The purpose of this investigation was to obtain information on the familial, genetic and social fate of these blind people.

Table I contains diagnoses of the 196 still available ex-pupils born between 1890 and 1952.

No pupils born prior to 1890 were alive. In the case of the younger ones, their life had not yet taken a definite course. Table I demonstrates that the causes of blindness are predominantly of hereditary origin. There were 81 corresponding to 2% of hereditary diseases as compared to only 18 corresponding to 8% of non-hereditary cases. Tapetoretinal degeneration and buphthalmia together accounted for nearly half of all hereditary cases of blindness.

This proves beyond any doubt the case for sensible genetic advice. However, it is essential, that we should first study the lives of past generations of blind people.

Table 2 shows that 115 out of 196 patients are unmarried. This corresponds to 60%.

The development in the respective age groups, as can be seen in this table, shows no definite trend toward more blind people marrying in modern times. However, the following facts give reason to assume that this

TABLE I

Katamnestic investigations in 196 former blind pupils (Blindenschule Ilvesheim)

Diagnosis	Number of pat.	%
Buphthalmus	44	22.5
Tapetoretinal Degeneration	35	17.9
Congenital Cataract	24	12.4
Mikrophthalmus	22	11.2
Ret. Detachment and Myopia maligna	14	7.1
Optic atrophy	14	7.1
Lawrence-Moon-Biedl Syndrome	2	1.0
Aniridia Cataracta pol. Myopia maligna	2	1.0
François' Syndrome Corneal dystrophy	1	0.5
Excessive Keratokonus	1	0.5
Hereditary diseases	159	81.2
Non hereditary diseases	37	18.8
	196	100

TABLE II

Social Statistics
Distribution of 115 unmarried blind persons

52♂			63♀	
Cities		62 : 53		Country side
25♂				27♂
37♀				26♀

Year of birth	Year of birth	Year of birth	Year of birth	Year of birth
1890-1912	1913-1922	1923-1932	1933-1942	1943-1952
25	18	21	27	24
5♂ : 19♀	8♂ : 10♀	6♂ : 10♀	15♂ : 12♀	17♂ : 7♀
	20♂ : 44♀		32♂ : 19♀	

situation will change:
1. Social assistance in the modern welfare is better organized. The risks inherent in such a marriage are, therefore, smaller.
2. The contact between blind and normal-vision people at their place of work is better — if one consider the present trend toward professions for blind people in office and industry — than in former times when they excelled mostly in handicraft activities.

Table 2 demonstrates that there are 52 blind unmarried men and 63 blind unmarried women. The unmarried women live mostly in urban communities. In rural districts blind girls have a better chance to marry. Here, in fact, the proportion is nearly equal: 27 men to 26 women.

The trend in the younger age groups seems to favor blind girls. As the statistics show the male-female ratio is reversed. However, it must be kept in mind, that as a rule girls marry younger than men. Therefore, from the last age group there are several men who will still get married. Cosmetic disfigurement plays a decisive role. Blind people suffering from tapetoretinal degeneration have relatively good marriage prospects; 86% of former pupils with visual handicaps such as mikrophthalmia remained single.

Social statistics on married blind people in Table III show the unfavorable position of blind girls compared to men. Sixty-eight blind men married as opposed to only 13 blind women. This is a ratio of 5 to 1.

TABLE III

Social Statistics
Distribution of 81 married persons

68♂ Cities		52 : 29	13♀ Country side	
	46♂/6♀			22♂/7♀
Year of birth	Year of birth	Year of birth	Year of birth	Year of birth
1890-1912	1913-1922	1923-1932	1933-1942	1943-1952
20	26	12	17	6
19♂ : 1♀	21♂ : 5♀	12♂ : 0♀	13♂ : 4♀	3♂ : 3♀
	52♂ : 6♀		16♂ : 7♀	

Urban environment seems to provide less favorable opportunities for blind girls than rural districts. In cities the ratio of blind married men to blind married women is 7.5 to 1, compared to 3 to 1 in rural areas.

More recently a trend emerged indicating that blind girls' chances of marriage are improving. However, if the modern welfare state continues to improve blind people's economic stability and likelihood of marriage, it is even more vital to provide pre-marital genetic advice. Useful information for such advice is provided by the life histories of blind married ex-pupils of the past decades.

The 81 blind married people in our katamnestic statistic have married in all 78 times. Several pupils from our school for the blind have intermarried. Refer to Table IV.

It is important to note that not one of these 78 marriages has been dissolved! The reason is due not only to the normal qualities of the partners, but also to financial and economic reasons which make the luxury of a divorce unlikely and unpractical. It must also be stressed that in these marriages affection and mutual dependence play a major role.

In 36 marriages, that is nearly half, there were no children. The marriage partners told us that in some cases they expressly intended not to have children out of a sense of responsibility. Only a small percentage is childless

TABLE IV

Katamnestic investigations in 196 former blind pupils (Blindenschule Ilvesheim)

115 stayed unmarried	
81 got married	= 78 marriages

Out of which	36 had no children
	36 had healthy children
	6 had blind children

as a result of sterilization of one of the partners carried out between 1933 and 1945.

Another 36 marriages, that is almost half of the group, have healthy children. Only 6 out of 78 marriages have one or more blind children.

This group is of particular significance. The question arises whether they should have been provided with premarital counseling.

Table V contains a breakdown of the 81 blind married ex-pupils.

TABLE V

Marriages of 81 blind former pupils

Out of which
20 married a blind partner
14♂ : 6♀
8 married a partially blind partner
4♂ : 4♀
53 married a partner with normal vision
50♂ : 3♀

The distribution of men and women shows that blind women have little chance to marry a man with normal vision. Whereas, in case of blind men the opposite is true. The ratio being 50 to 3. In the case of marriages blind to blind to partial vision this ratio improves.

For this reason blind to blind and blind to partial vision marriages can never be avoided. Added to this is the fact that opportunities for blind people to come into contact with normal sighted people are few, whereas blind people meet and get to know each other in schools for the blind, rehabilitation centers and within their own organization. Our katamnestic investigations have shown that nearly all blind to blind and blind to partial vision marriages resulted from contacts made in these areas.

Table VI shows a survey of 20 blind people who are married to a blind partner.

Of these marriages, 10 are childless, representing over 50%. In case of blind to partially blind marriages exactly half are childless, and in case of blind to normal vision marriages less than half are childless.

Six of these 17 marriages have healthy children, one couple has one blind child.

TABLE VI

Marriage Blind/Blind
Out of 196 former blind pupils (Blindenschule Ilvesheim)

---

20 married a blind partner = 17 marriages

Out of which   10 had no children
6 had healthy children
1 had blind children

Table VII shows that in 6 marriages all with healthy children — with the exception of one marriage, where the case of blindness was unknown — one partner lost the vision due to a non-hereditary cause.

TABLE VII

Marriage Blind/Blind
6 marriages with healthy offspring

Diagnosis	Diagnosis	Number of children
Buphthalmus ♀	Postblennorheic leucoma cornea ♂	1♂
Buphthalmus ♂	(Amaurosis of unknown cause ♀)	2♂ 2♀
Ret. Detachment Myopia maligna ♂	(Leucoma after lime-burn ♀)	1♂
Congen. Cataract ♀	Optic atrophy after meningitis ♂	2♂
Tapetoretinal Degeneration ♂	(Postttraumatic optic atrophy ♀)	2♂
Leucoma after lime-burn ♂	(Congen. Cataract ♀)	1♂

From the genetic point of view and even with the most careful advice there could have been no possible reason for objecting to these marriages, especially since the other blind partner was afflicted with a disease in which a recessive mode of inheritance is very probable.

As a rule buphthalmia (pedigree 1) and tapetoretinal degeneration (pedigree 2) are inherited as a recessive trait.

Even the presence of blindness in several siblings, as for example in the pedigree of tapetoretinal degeneration, would not be a valid reason for objecting to a childless marriage. In fact, the marriage of one of the four afflicted sons had produced no blind offsprings.

The existence of tapetoretinal degeneration in two successive generations can be considered a pseudo-dominant trait — if one assumes the presence of consanguinity. In the case of one of our families (pedigree 3) this has been confirmed, neither of the two children is blind.

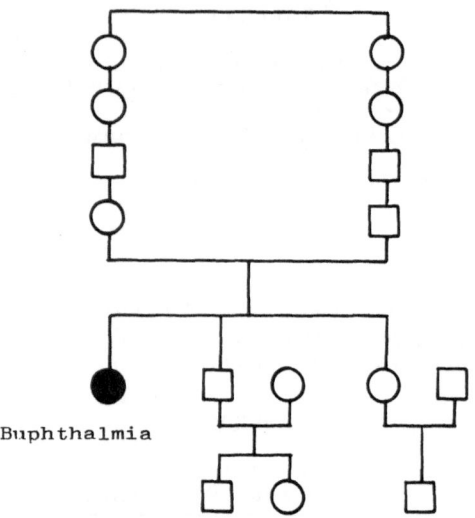

Buphthalmia

Pedigree (1) of S.M. (born 1937)
Recessive hereditary in the case of Buphthalmia.
Consanguinity.

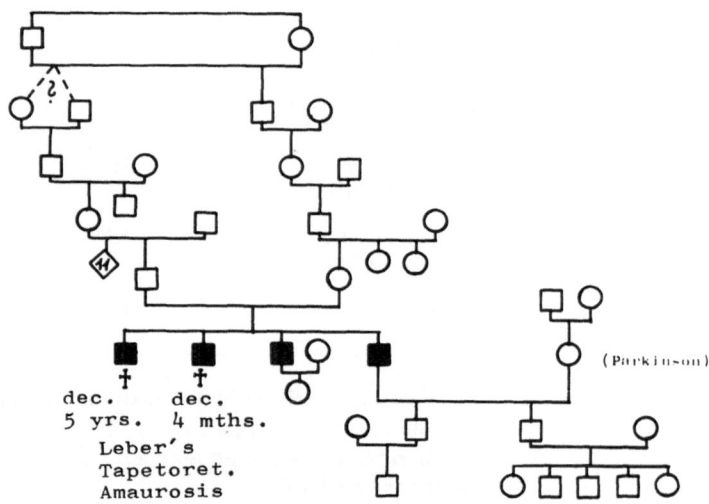

(Parkinson)

dec.   dec.
5 yrs.   4 mths.

Leber's
Tapetoret.
Amaurosis

Pedigree (2) of E.L. (born 1901)
Reccessive hereditary disease – Normal.
Consanguinity.

In case of relatively frequent hereditary disorders such as buphthalmia and tapetoretinal degeneration there is of course always a possibility, however small, that the partner might be a heterozygote of precisely this disease. Thus can be explained the tragic fate of one of the blind to blind families which had a blind child: The father had buphthalmia, the mother dominant cataracta congenita, and the child had both buphthalmia and cataracta con-

66

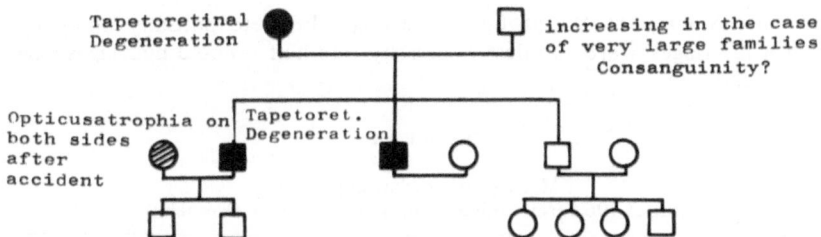

Pedigree (3) of E.K. (born 1937)
Pseudo-dominance in the case of recessive hereditary disease and blindness resulting from accident.

TABLE VIII

Marriage Blind/Blind

1 marriage with one blind offspring

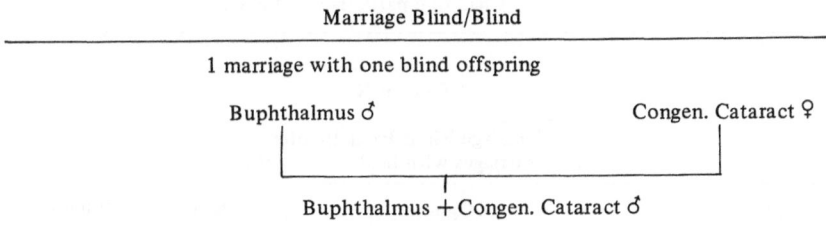

genita. Refer to Table VIII.

The complete pedigree (4) shows that the cataracta congenita, being a dominant form, was to be expected with 50% probability; Buphthalmia was not expected.

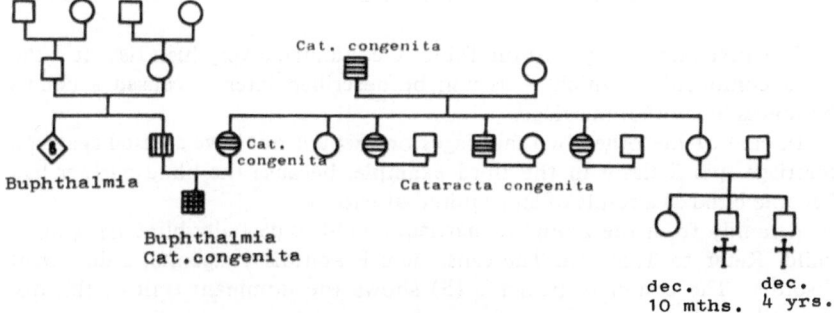

Pedigree (4) of W.Sp. (born 1969)
Combination of recessive and dominant hereditary disease.

The mother of the young blind patient must have been a carrier not only of the dominant gene of cataracta congenita, but also a carrier of the buphthalmia gene. This could not have been predicted. In genetic guidance one would probably have advised against having children from this marriage, because of buphthalmia. What caused the blindness, though, was buphthalmia and not the cataract which in itself could have been removed by surgery.

67

Table IX contains the group of marriages blind to partially blind. Of these 8 marriages 4 are childless — exactly one half — and 3 marriages have healthy children.

TABLE IX

Marriage Blind/Partially blind
Out of 196 former blind pupils (Blindenschule Ilvesheim)

---

8 married a visually handicapped person
= 8 marriages

Out of which

4 had no children
3 had healthy children
1 had one partially blind child

TABLE X

Marriage Blind/Partially blind
3 marriages with healthy offspring

Diagnosis	Diagnosis	Number of Children
Congen. Cataract ♀	(Aniridia ♂)	1♀
Tapetoret. Degeneration ♀	(Congen. Cataract ♂)	1♀ 1♂
OD total Leucoma ♂ OS Anophthalmus (after German measles)	(Congen. Cataract ♀)	2♂

The first marriage shown on Table X contained a very high risk. It is the same combination which — as will be described later — caused a child's blindness in another marriage.

In case of the other two marriages one would not have advised against a marriage, particularly in the third example, because the blind partner had become blind as a result of an acquired disease.

A family from the group of marriages blind to partially blind has a blind child. Refer to Table XI. The cause here is aniridia congenita, a dominant disorder. The complete pedigree (5) shows the dominant trait of this disorder through 3 generations.

The last and largest group consists of 53 blind to normal vision marriages. As can be seen in Table XII, 22 of these marriages had no children. This is less than half, as compared to the two other groups.

The marriages illustrated in Table XIII with healthy children confirm what has already been said: 8 blind people have lost their vision due to non-hereditary diseases. Genetically speaking there was no risk in their case.

Of the other blind people, 8 had tapetoretinal degeneration and 5 buphthalmia, both recessive hereditary disorders. Despite a relatively high number of children in these marriages there are no blind children.

TABLE XI

Marriage Blind/Partially blind

1 Marriage with 1 healthy child
and 1 partially blind child

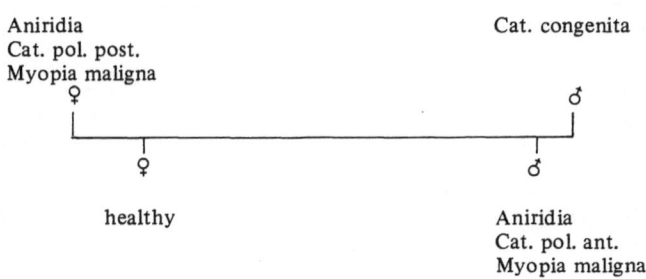

Aniridia
Cat. pol. post.
Myopia maligna
♀

Cat. congenita
♂

♀
healthy

♂
Aniridia
Cat. pol. ant.
Myopia maligna

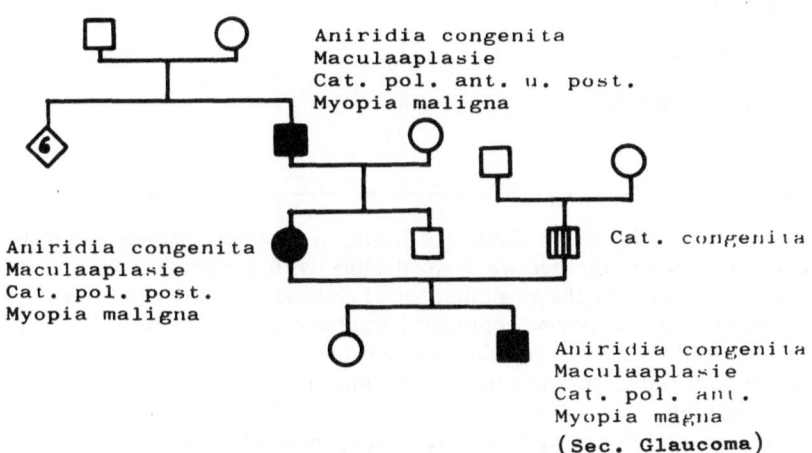

Aniridia congenita
Maculaaplasie
Cat. pol. ant. u. post.
Myopia maligna

Aniridia congenita
Maculaaplasie
Cat. pol. post.
Myopia maligna

Cat. congenita

Aniridia congenita
Maculaaplasie
Cat. pol. ant.
Myopia magna
(Sec. Glaucoma)

Pedigree (5) of U.K. (born 1969)
Dominant hereditary disease.

TABLE XII

Marriage Blind/Normal vision
Out of 196 former blind pupils (Blindenschule Ilvesheim)

53 (50♂, 3♀) married
a partner with normal vision = 53 marriages

Out of which

22 had no offspring
27 had healthy children
4 had blind children

TABLE XIII

Marriage Blind/Normal vision
27 marriages with healthy offspring

Diagnosis	Number of patients	Number of children
Tapetoretinal degeneration	8	3 x 1 4 x 2 1 x 5
Buphthalmus	5	2 x 1 1 x 2 2 x 3
Congen. Cataract	2	1 x 2 1 x 6
Optic atrophies (1 by turricephalus)	2	1 x 1 1 x 2
Ret. Detachment Myopia maligna	1	1 x 2
Mikrophthalmus	1	1 x 1
Non hereditary diseases	8	3 x 1 3 x 2 1 x 3 1 x 6

In marriages with fewer children suffering from other diseases it is difficult to determine whether we were dealing with a recessive disorder or whether as a result of the small number of children, no blind child was born in marriages with otherwise dominant hereditary disorders. From the diagnostic point of view either possibility is feasible.

Table XIV shows that in a blind to normal vision marriage blind children are also possible.

Four out of 53 marriages from this group have blind children. Here we find 2 dominant disorders — aniridia and the François-syndrome type. The two diseases probably represent a form of dominance.

If one compares the possibility of giving birth to a blind child, in the case of blind to blind and blind to partially blind marriages on the one hand, and in the case of blind to normal vision marriages on the other, the differences are not as great as one might at first suppose.

In 25 marriages blind to blind and blind to partially blind, two blind children were born. In 53 marriages blind to normal vision 4 blind were born. Refer to Table XV.

Blind to blind marriages cannot be avoided, by virtue of the fact that blind girls have a greater chance to get married. At the same time, it is encouraging to see that dispositions towards diseases in these marriages is not much greater than in blind to normal vision marriages. Marriages between two blind partners will in all likelihood increase in the future.

The last table (XVI) shows the professional situation of blind people. It

70

TABLE XIV

Marriage Blind/Normal vision
4 marriages, which had blind children

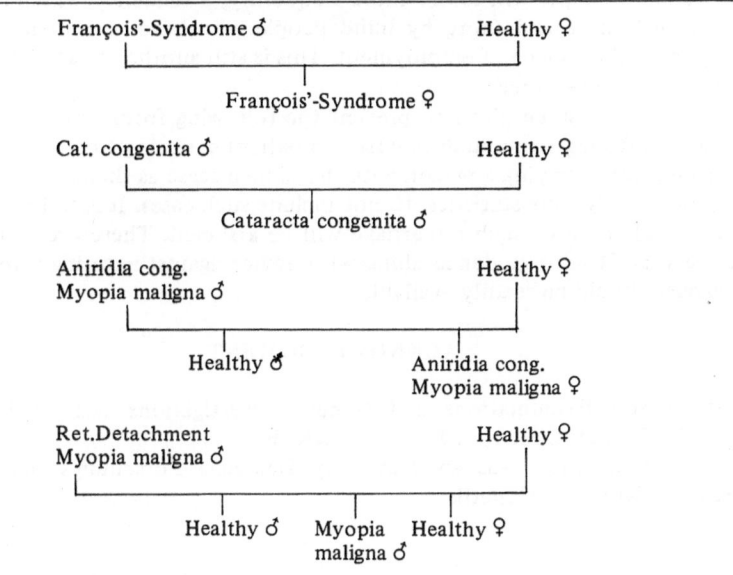

TABLE XV

Marriages of 81 blind former pupils = 78 marriages

Marriages	Total of marriages	Marriages with blind children
Blind/Blind Blind/Partially blind	25	2
Blind/Normal vision	53	4

TABLE XVI

Social Statistics

Year of birth	Handicraft professions	Changing to another profession	Profession in office	Changing to another profession
1890-1912	38	10	1	–
1913-1922	40	19	1	–
1923-1932	30	20	1	–
1933-1942	34	22	9	–
1943-1952	16	7	13	1 (Computer specialist)

can be seen that handicraft professions are not as popular and that they are being abandoned. On the other hand positions in offices and industry are on the increase, thus improving the possibilities for more personal contact. As a result blind people will marry more frequently, a tendency which has been confirmed more and more by blind people who have met their marriage partner at their place of employment. This is still another reason for genetic advice to be intensified.

Warning must be given to prevent the following from arising: that of a patient suffering from buphthalmia or a patient suffering from tapetoretinal degeneration marrying a person with the same disease as theirs.

Fortunately, our statistics do not include such cases. It is to be expected that all children of such a marriage will be afflicted. Therefore, it is imperative that genetic guidance along with advice against entering into such a marriage should be readily available.

ACKNOWLEDGMENT

Katamnestic Examinations and Genetic investigations were assisted by APPEL, CH., DELUIGI, S. & LOHMANN, E.

The publication was sponsored by Deutsche Forschungsgemeinschaft (SFB 35 'Klinische Genetik').

INCIDENCE OF IMPAIRED VISION DUE TO
REFRACTIVE ERRORS AMONG COLLEGE STUDENTS
OF CALCUTTA

RANABIR MUKHERJI

(Calcutta, India)

Uncorrected refractive errors can give rise to considerable visual impairement which may become permanent. Measurements of visual acuity and ocular refraction are, therefore, important. A study of visual acuity helps in the assessment of the requirements for ophthalmic care in an entire community. The incidence of impaired vision due to refractive errors among young college students in Calcutta was studied during 1970-71.

There were approximately 15,000 students enrolled in three universities in Calcutta. From this group an unselected sample of 1,528 were randomly selected. They ranged from 16 to 26 years of age. The visual acuity of each eye was tested separately.

Squints were noted by the cover test. Retinoscopy under cycloplegia was done. The visual acuity after correction with glasses was noted. Those with pathologic findings such as corneal and lens opacities, choroidal and retinal diseases and the like were excluded.

Normal visual acuity of 6/6 was noted in 70.3 percent of the students: the vision of 25.2 percent of the students could be restored to normal with corrective glasses. This left 4.5 percent of the group where normal vision could not be achieved with glasses. In 2.6 percent of the cases, visual acuity was 6/18 or less.

Fifty-eight students — 3.8 percent — had squint. Forty-six of these were unilateral and 43 convergent. Divergent squint was present in 15 cases; alternating squint in 12 cases.

Among 58 students with squint, 46 were amblyopic in the squinting eye. In 40 students, vision in the amblyopic eye was 6/18 or less, corresponding in 2.6 percent.

In this study, the extent of impaired vision — less than 6/9 — among college students of Calcutta due to refractive errors was found to be 77 percent. Good visual acuity could be attained in 96 percent students after correction of refractive errors. This study compares favorably to that of PARNELL (1951) among Oxford undergraduates in 1951. PARNELL found 64 percent good vision in male and 59.1 percent good vision in female students. However, the total number of students he studied included only 279 men and 170 women. Twenty percent of the Oxford students had vision of 6/36 or less.

SORSBY and his co-workers in 1960 found visual acuity to be normal in over 80 percent of young males. Only 0.4 percent of this group had visual acuity of 6/18 or less.

The incidence of 3.8 percent squint in the student population of Calcutta that we examined is high. SORSBY, in a series of 1,033 young men, found the incidence of squint to be only 4.0 percent. Amblyopia ex anopsia occurred in only 0.5 percent of SORSBY'S cases. On the other hand, we found 1.2 percent of severe amblyopia with vision of 6/36 or less. It is of interest to note that more than one among 100 college students in Calcutta had no useful vision in one eye due to squint resulting mostly from uncorrected errors of refraction.

CONCLUSION

A study on the incidence of impaired vision due to refractive errors among 1,528 college students in three universities of Calcutta was made. The extent of impaired vision – less than 6/9 – due to refractive errors was found to be 23.6 percent, and good vision – 6/9 or more – could be attained in 96 percent after correction. The incidence of squint and amblyopia due to refractive errors was found to be 3.8 percent and 1.2 percent, respectively.

REFERENCES

PARNELL, R.W. *Brit. J. Ophthal.*, 35: *467* (1951).
SORSBY, A., SHERIDAN, M., LEARY, G.A. & BENJAMIN, B. *Brit. Med. J.*, 1: *1394* (1960).

CLASSIFICATION OF XEROPHTHALMIA

K.H. TENG

(Bandung, Indonesia)

Xerophthalmia is caused by vitamin A deficiency. It is characterized by dryness of the conjunctiva and often of the cornea. Blindness may be prevented by the administration of large doses of vitamin A.

Nightblindness is a frequent early symptom. Because of its subjective nature it is of little help in classification, treatment and prognosis of the disease.

Bitot's spots are found in about 75% of xerophthalmic children, and in some adults.

The underlying social economic causes of Xerophthalmia are poverty, nutritional ignorance, and neglect by the parents. Gastrointestinal and metabolic diseases frequently accompany the condition. The diet and childhood diseases differ from country to country. To some extent so does Xerophthalmia.

Laboratory examinations are impractical on a mass scale for the early detection of vitamin A deficiency.

Clinical findings in Xerophthalmia include: Bitot spots, pigmentation of the bulbar conjunctiva, decreased elasticity and wrinkling of the conjunctiva, elongated eyelashes, prominence of the pores of the Meibomian glands ducts at the lid margins, the xerophthalmic fundus, and Xerosis of the cornea.

I should like to propose the following classification:

First stage: Xerophthalmia with no corneal involvement, and good prognosis.

Second stage: Corneal involvement, which may be reversible.

Third stage: Corneal involvement with scar formations that are irreversible.

This classification serves well in clinical practice. Paramedical personnel are able to distinguish between patients who may be treated on an ambulatory basis and those who need hospital care.

Keratomalacia may occur suddenly with or without xerosis, following a febrile disease. Classification of Xerophthalmia into three stages enables the clinican to assess the severity of the disease and employ appropriate methods of therapy.

HYPOVITAMINOSIS A FROM INTESTINAL INFESTATIONS

I.S. ROY & E. AHMED

(Calcutta, India)

The normal need of vitamin A varies according to age, state of health and general demands of the body. Manifestations of hypovitaminosis A become evident when the average daily consumption is less than half of the recommended dose. The ocular signs can be readily detected. Hence routine examination of the conjunctiva and cornea of every child who attends a clinic is highly recommended.

In India, keratomalacia is the commonest cause of pediatric blindness. In 4.39 million blind children in India, about 40 percent were blind due to keratomalacia (VENKATASWAMY, 1966).

The incidence of hypovitaminosis A in all likelihood is higher than what has been documented by various world surveys.

According to RODGER & SINCLAIR, (1969) stores of vitamin A in the liver should last for nearly a year, but the deficiency may be precipitated by defective absorption, defective storage or excessive loss of the vitamin. A complex relationship exists between hypovitaminosis A and protein deficiency.

In our opinion, defective absorption appears to be the most significant contributory factor in the causation of hypovitaminosis A. The relationship of the condition with intestinal worms has not been fully established. TIWAR (1962, 1966) from India reported the presence of intestinal worms in 95 percent of 1,500 cases of keratomalacia. AHMED & ROY in 1970 found worms in 50 percent of the cases. They included Entamoeba histolytica, giardia, round worm and hook worm.

Stool examinations at intermittent intervals are likely to reveal ova, parasites or cysts. SINHA (1966) believes that medications are poorly absorbed in the presence of severe diarrhea.

In 1971, during the last massive influx of refugees from Bangladesh, we examined a great many patients with hypovitaminosis A. Thirty percent of the children in the refugee camp showed evidence of hypovitaminosis A with early ocular signs. They were treated with both vitamin A and anthelmintics. None of them developed keratomalacia.

From our clinical experience on large numbers of cases, we recommend the administration of vitamin A along with supplementary measures and the use of anthelmintics.

REFERENCES

AHMED, E. & ROY, S.N. Ocular Signs of Hypovitaminosis A and Intestinal Infections. *Indian Pract.*, 23: *225-226* (1970).

RODGER, F.C. & SINCLAIR, H.M. in: Metabolic and Nutritional Eye Diseases. Thomas, U.S.A., p. 187, 1969.

SINHA, B.N. Influence of Protein on Keratomalacia. *J. Indian M.A.*, 47: *55* (1966).

TIWARY, R. Ocular Manifestations of Intestinal Worms Infestation. XIX Int. Congress Ophthal., New Delhi, *Acta* I: *(1962)*.

TIWARY, R. Intestinal Infections and Ocular Lesions With Particular Reference to Keratomalacia, *J. All India Opth. Soc.*, 14: *87-88* (1966).

VENKATASWAMY, G. Malnutritional Blindness in India, *J. Indian M.A.*, 47: *67* (1966).

PROPHYLACTIC USE OF VITAMIN A IN NUTRITIONAL EYE DISEASE

P. SIVA REDDY

(Hyderabad, India)

The rational approach for prevention of vitamin A deficiency in children consists of improvement of their diets. Prophylactic therapy should be instituted in areas where diets are deficient. It has been estimated that in India 4% children between the age of 6 months and 5 years become visually handicapped.

Prophylactic measures against malnutrition and its effect on the eyes are carried out by the National Institute of Nutrition, Hyderabad. Over 2,000 children between the ages of 6 months and 5 years were given a single oral dose of 100,000 I.U. of vitamin A once a year. The results of this study in 1969 showed that a single annual oral dose of vitamin A can maintain serum vitamin A levels at a satisfactory level for a period of 6 months, or even longer. From a biochemical standpoint this is an important observation. From a clinical standpoint it has been observed that a small percentage of cases developed signs of acute toxicity due to vitamin A.

In 1970, deficiency eye disease numbered 3,496; in 1971, 3,636; in 1972, 3,910; and in 1973, 3,236. Sixty to sixty-five percent of the cases came from rural areas and the lower Socio-economic strata of society. During a 4-year period, we examined 334,034 patients. Of this group, 12,780 were caused by malnutrition. Despite prophylactic vitamin A therapy, attendance of nutritionally deficient children with eye diseases has not decreased! Our clinical study revealed that 50% of xerosis of the conjunctiva occurs between the 6-12 year age group; 40% occurs in the 3-5 year age group. Corneal xerosis occurs most often between 6 months to 2 years.

In 70% of patients between 3-10 years of age, nightblindness was due to vitamin A deficiency. Bitots spots were found to be common in the 5-10 year age group. Seventy percent of xerophthalmia cases occurred in the 3-10 year age group.

After correlating results of field trials of oral single massive Vitamin A administration with patients attending Sarojini Devi Eye Hospital and Institute of Ophthalmology, we doubt the value of massive vitamin A therapy alone as preventive factor in xerosis and keratomalacia. The probable coexistence of protein-calorie malnutrition, along with various B Complex deficiencies, may be responsible.

NUTRITION REHABILITATION CENTER, DEPARTMENTS OF OPHTHALMOLOGY & PAEDIATRICS, GOVERNMENT ERSKINE HOSPITAL, MADURAI, S. INDIA

G. VENKATASWAMY, K.A. KRISHNAMURTHY, P. CHANDRA & S.A. KABIR

(Madurai, India)

NUTRITION REHABILITATION CENTER

Since 1956 large numbers of patients with eye signs of Vitamin A and B deficiency were studied in the Eye Department of the Government Erskine Hospital, Madurai, India.

TABLE I

Diagnosis	Number of cases seen during						
	1967	1968	1969	1970	1971	1972	1973
Night blindness	31	51	117	83	43	143	160
Xerosis	505	369	412	502	377	543	645
Bitot's spots	453	489	725	630	569	520	693
Congenital pigmentation	109	115	56	18	53	58	35
Keratomalacia	240	216	245	313	220	142	118

The principal aim of the Nutritional Rehabilitation Center is to educate mothers to improve the nutritional status of their children and prevent blindness. Locally available foods are given to the children at a cost their parents can afford. Children attending the Ophthalmic and Paediatric Out-Patient Departments of the Government Erskine Hospital, Madurai, with ocular eye signs of vitamin deficiencies are admitted to the Center. The children are accompanied by their mothers, grandmothers or sisters or some other relative. A cook is employed in the Center. Food is prepared and distributed to the children. Those children who come from nearby or distant villages are admitted to stay for a fortnight at the Center. At the time when children are admitted, records are maintained on their nutritional status, eye sight, intercurrent diseases, fevers, diarrhea, and other pertinent medical problems.

When the mothers are convinced that the diet had improved their children, the children are discharged. It was often difficult to persuade mothers to remain with their children for one or two weeks as they had other children to look after in their homes or other duties to attend to. From the beginning, the mothers were given duties to go to the market, choose the green leafy vegetables, cook and also to distribute food. Those children who had their treatment in the Nutrition Rehabilitation Center were followed and their progress recorded. Table II illustrates the number of children fed during the last three years for malnutritional diseases.

TABLE II

Age Group	Grade I	Grade II	Grade III	Total
0 - 1	–	–	5	5
1 - 2	4	8	103	115
2 - 3	4	29	186	219
3 - 4	2	34	156	219
4 - 5	2	17	70	89
5 - & Above	–	10	36	46
Total	12	98	556	666

TABLE III

Age group	X_0	X_1	X_2	$X_{3}a$	$X_{3}b$	X_4	Total
0 - 1	–	2	1	2	–	–	5
1 - 2	6	44	8	13	6	3	80
2 - 3	13	80	21	38	9	3	164
3 - 4	9	83	27	27	10	3	159
4 - 5	2	47	11	12	6	2	80
5 & above	1	22	8	7	2	1	41
Total	31	278	76	99	33	12	529

Most of the children were brought to the Center in a bad state with Grade III or IV malnutrition and complications that included diarrhea, fever, and other illnesses. The mothers usually gave quack treatment or home remedies before they brought their children to the hospital. They generally did not attach importance to night blindness or weight loss. Magic cures, talismans and quack remedies, such as removing foreign bodies from intestines, herbal treatment, and the like had been administered prior to hospitalization. Children who are actually ill are admitted as in-patients and the other children are treated as out-patients. In both the places, i.e., in Wards and Out-Patient Department in the hospital, there is no way of educating the mothers to understand the nature and causes of the children's ailment and ways it can be cured. In the Nutrition Rehabilitation Center, emphasis is on education and practical demonstrations to mothers as well as the improvement of the nutritional status by proper feeding. The Center is located in the hospital. It was not easily possible for the mothers to differentiate between the Center and the hospital. Quite a high percentage of mothers are convinced now that the food given to the children is good and upon discharge from the Center they follow the same diet in their own homes.

RESULTS OF THE FEEDING AND TREATMENT

Of 666 children at the Center during the past three years, 73 died, 144 had keratomalacia, 15 lost all their vision in both eyes and 41 had partial loss of vision in both eyes, and 33 had lost the vision in one eye. Children with night blindness and angular stomatitis became completely cured.

FOLLOW-UP

Children who left the Center were followed-up at 14-day intervals. Their mothers were helpful in encouraging other mothers who attended the Center and our staff visited the homes of the mothers and children who attended the Center and followed their progress. In this manner, mothers were educated and the children's nutritional status and health condition were recorded.

TRAINING OF CHILD CARE WORKERS

The Government of Tamil Nadu made provisions for the establishment of village nutrition centers in two community blocks near Madurai. The Associated Countrywomen of the World financed village nutrition centers in one block near Madurai. For all of these, we trained child care workers. Training at the Nutrition Rehabilitation Center in Madurai includes demonstration of proper feeding. Much time is spent to educate staff for the assessment of nutritional status, recognition signs of malnutrition, proper treatment and feeding. Child care workers keep records of children under their supervision. They are also taught to recognize the common diseases of children and methods to prevent them.

TRAINING OF APPLIED NUTRITION PROGRAMS, STAFF AND OTHER STAFF

Most of the people do not have a definite idea of the problem of malnutrition existing in preschool children. They have no practical experience of the immensity of the problem and ways of solving the problem.

NUTRITION EDUCATION

We prepared a Guide Book for Child Care Workers in local Tamil language. Nutrition education posters have been devised and printed, various pamphlets have been written, films have been made to show nutritional status of the children and the work of the Nutrition Rehabilitation Center. Slides have been prepared for educating the public.

DISCUSSION

Most mothers had very little idea of proper nutrition and growth of children. They believe that rich people look better than the poor. They are not aware of the common cause of infections and methods to prevent them.

Therefore, many of the children are treated with quack remedies. Quack remedies are looked upon as a magic method. After finding such remedies are futile, parents bring their children to the hospital when severe malnutritional diseases and infections develop. If the people became aware of the causes of these diseases and they were educated to prevent them, most of the misery can be avoided in the country. In the Eye Department of the Government Erskine Hospital, Madurai, nearly 50 percent of the patients attending suffer from infections due to malnutrition. The children attending the Nutrition Rehabilitation Center are examined carefully by the Child Care Workers assisted by a part-time ophthalmologist and part-time paediatrician. A separate file is maintained for each child. Children are fed in the Center. The results of the feeding in the Center show that there is great increase in weights even in 15 days time. Early eye signs of corneal Xerosis are clear in several cases and the mothers are convinced that the food given to their children in the Nutrition Rehabilitation Center has helped their children. By educating all the mothers, we have been able to prepare films, posters, books, pamphlets, slides, etc.

Apart from educating the mothers, we have conducted nutrition courses in our Nutrition Rehabilitation Center to several categories of Tamil Nadu Government staff.

In the Wards and in the Out-Patient Department, individual attention is not given to each child's feeding. Most of these children have poor appetites and it takes at least 8 to 10 days to persuade them to eat and develop appetite. Each child in the Nutrition Rehabilitation Center is carefully watched where the child is taking its feeds and with patience, children are persuaded to eat small quantities until their appetites improve.

Nutrients provided from the menu for in-patients

Nutrients	Quantity
Calories	1369
Protein	51.1 gm.
Calcium	1.034 gm.
Iron	25.9 mg.
Vitamin A (Carotene)	4624.04 mg.

Nutrients provided from the menu for out-patients

Nutrients	Quantity
Calories	949
Protein	35.06 g.
Calcium	1.0 g.
Iron	16.29 mg.
Vitamin A (Carotene)	4006 mg.

OCULAR TRAUMA IN JAPAN

AKIRA NAKAJIMA & YOSHINAO FUKADO

(Tokyo & Kawasaki, Japan)

Ocular trauma caused by accidents is theoretically preventable. In actual fact, prevention is not easy.

Table I indicates the number of accidents and consequent permanent visual impairment that occurred in school. During 1970-1972, 164 eyes were severely damaged by accidents. This represents one-fourth of the total cases of permanent functional damage.

TABLE I

Number of Accidents at School (1972)

	Students	Accidents	Percentage
Primary School (6-12 yrs old)	9,500,000	300,712	3.07
	4,720,000	222,604	4.72

Permanent visual impairment during 1970-72: 164 eyes
Approximately 3 cases per million students per year.

Table II illustrates that in over 60 percent of the cases, something flew into the eyes. Fortunately, none of them were binocular, and none of the children became blind. Approximately three eyes per one million students were lost or severely damaged each year. It would be difficult to further reduce this rate.

TABLE II

Causes of Ocular Trauma at School

Cause	Primary	Secondary	Total	Percentage
Flying objects	39	62	101	61.5
Direct injuries	30	13	43	26.2
Other causes	11	9	20	22.3
Total	80	84	164	

None of this group had binocular blindness.
Approximately 3 eyes were injured each year per one million students.

Table III summarizes industrial accidents in Japan. Among thirty million industrial workers, nearly two million accidents occurred during 1969. The majority of these minor accidents. Five hundred thousand of the injured needed more than four days to recover. Permanent damage or disability resulted in eighty thousand workers. Two percent had eye injuries.

TABLE III

Eye Injury in Industry (Japan, 1969)

Industrial workers	33,250,000	
Industrial accidents	1,715,000	
Absent for less than 3 days	1,213,930	eye injuries
Absent for more than 4 days	495,616	10,885 (2.2%)
Permanent disability	79,579	2,254 (2.8%)
Death	5,460	

Table IV shows the type of industry and eye injury. Mining was by far the most dangerous industry capable of producing eye injuries. Nearly one in a hundred workers had some eye injury per year. However, most of them were slight and only one-tenth had permanent partial disability. Contruction and forestry ranked high in causing eye injuries.

TABLE IV

Type of Industry and Eye Injury

Type of Industry	Workers	Eye Injury	Rate (10^{-4})	Permanent Damage	Rate
Manufacture	13,250,000	4,750	3.6	1,098	0.8
Construction	3,400,000	2,423	7.1	650	2.0
Mining	235,000	1,737	73.9	151	6.4
Transportation	185,000	712	3.8	105	0.6
Forestry	327,000	633	9.4	83	1.2
Others	15,853,000	1,895	1.3	167	0.1
Total	33,250,000	10,885	3.3	2,254	0.7

Trauma by hitting the eye by flying objects was the most frequent cause. Nearly half of the industrial eye injuries were either corneal abrasions or foreign bodies, but perforating wounds occurred in nearly 40 percent of all cases.

Table V illustrates that among approximately ten thousand patients, one-tenth had visual acuity of 0.1 or less in one or both eyes. Half of the injured eyes were caused by trauma. Only three percent had binocular involvement. The total number of industrial accidents is decreasing.

In the United States, since 1973 all eyeglasses must be shatter-proof. A survey in Japan revealed only a few eye injuries caused by broken eyeglasses.

Table VI was compiled from inquiries sent to five thousand Japanese ophthalmologists. Replies were received from 25 percent of this group.

TABLE V

Visual Acuity Among Patients in Kanto Rosai Hospital (1970-73)

Vision in one eye 0.1 or less	1,114 (10%)
Trauma	519 (5%)
Binocular	15 (2.8%)
Total number of patients	10,973

TABLE VI

Eye Injuries as Related to Eyeglasses or Contact Lenses
Result of Inquiry from all Ophthalmologists in Japan (1972)

Inquiry sent to	4760 eye specialists	
Replies received from	1173 (24.6%)	181 hospitals
		992 clinics

They were asked if they noted permanent impairment of vision caused by eyeglass breakage or contact lens wear. In all, 91 cases were reported by over one thousand ophthalmologists. Out of these, 47 had vision over 0.4 or better, and less than half had vision 0.3 or less. The majority of patients were injured while working, driving or participating in sports. Most of them were male in their teens or twenties. In only two were both eyes damaged.

Visual impairment caused by contact lens wear occurred in 33 cases. Among them, only 12 cases had vision of 0.3 or less. five were caused by trauma while wearing contact lenses.

TABLE VII

Estimated Incidence of Trauma
as a Result of The Use of Eyeglasses During 1972

100-400, vision 0.3 or lower; 50-170
eyeglass wearers in Japan: 30,000,000
incidence: 10^{-5}

Visual impairment by contact lens wear:
30-120, vision 0.3 or less; 7-30
contact lens wearers in Japan: 2,000,000
incidence: ca. 10^{-5}

Incidence of Purulent Corneal Ulcer (1970)

Result of inquiry study from 2,105 ophthalmologists
in Japan.

3-10 per 10^5 per year (cause: corneal trauma 60%,
foreign body 20%,
others 20%)

Table VII shows the estimated incidence of occular damage caused by eyeglass or contact lens wear. This is of the order of one in one hundred thousand. As a result, Japan decided not to follow the regulation of the United States Food and Drug Administration in requiring mandatory safety eyeglass lenses for all.

Minor corneal trauma followed by infection may lead to loss of an eye. A survey in Japan on the incidence of purulent corneal ulcer revealed 3 to 10 cases of infected corneal ulcers per one hundred thousand per year. Proper first aid and medical care for minor corneal trauma is important. Health education of the public in Japan about possible dangers of corneal abrasions has resulted in the low prevalence of this complication.

Prevention of ocular trauma and injury requires careful analysis and control of all possible risk factors. There is no royal road for the prevention of ocular trauma!

PREVENTION OF OCULAR INJURIES

J.D.C. MACDIARMID

(Hamilton, New Zealand)

INTRODUCTION

Before discussing methods of preventing injuries to the eye and subsequent loss of vision one must review the most common causes and then decide upon the most effective methods of eliminating or preventing such accidents.

CAUSES OF OCULAR TRAUMA

During the calendar year 1968 the New Zealand Society for the Prevention of Blindness conducted a nationwide survey of all major ocular injuries. This was done by presenting a standard request card in a prepaid envelope, to all ophthalmologists in the country with a request that they notify all injuries in which loss of vision in one or other eye to some degree was sustained as a result of that injury.

Table I shows that 482 such injuries were reported in one calendar year. These were reported by 52 ophthalmologists from a population of almost 3 million people. Returns from some areas were lower than would be anticipated considering returns from other areas and therefore the incidence could possibly be in excess of 500. It is also shown that 164 of these injuries occurred in people under the age of 16; 94 were under the age of 10.

TABLE I

Ocular Injuries Causing Loss of Sight

(12 month period. N.Z. Society Prevention Blindness)		
482	TOTAL	
164	BELOW	16 yrs.
94	BELOW	10 yrs.

Table II illustrates a breakdown of where such injuries occurred. By far the most site, 43.6%, is at home. The next most common being industrial, followed by farming, sporting, motor vehicle accidents. The school laboratory took only a minor place.

TABLE II

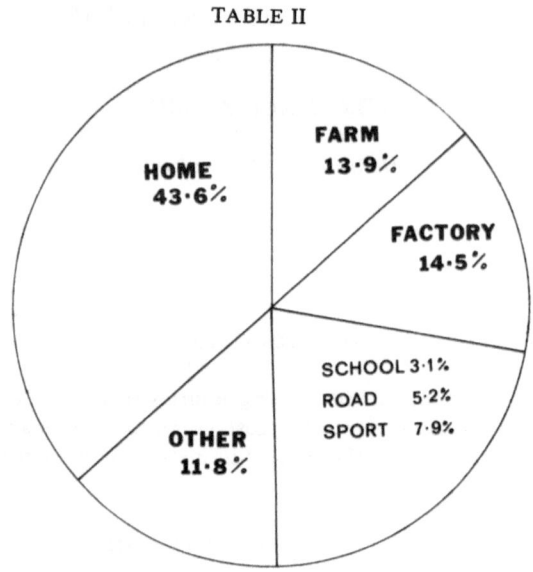

OCULAR INJURIES CAUSING LOSS OF SIGHT

(N.Z. 12mth. PERIOD)

INDUSTRIAL INJURIES

Statistics produced by our Department of Labour are provided in a different way. They represent injured workers who had some time off work, most of them being away from work for less than one week and not causing significant visual loss. The Labour Department however was more concerned with loss of time from industry rather than damage to eyesight.

Table III shows the causative agent, the most common cause being foreign body in the eye followed by burns and scalds and lacerations.

Table IV shows that foreign bodies were usually caused by a piece flying from a hand tool, from machinery or miscellaneous flying articles, dust, etc. In this review one statistic emerged that was important. Table V shows that by far the greatest number of these injuries either welding or grinding occurred in the hours 7 pm or 8 pm of the working day and these tend to reflect that towards the end of the day, when people have become tired they tend to be somewhat careless about safety measures.

453 such accidents were investigated by departmental inspectors. It was found that in 93 no protective device had been provided; in 191 the proper protective device had been provided but had not been worn at the time; in 46 cases the fit of the protection had not been properly adjusted; 27 had the wrong device for the purpose; 15 showed a lack of maintenance and in 54 there was an adequate protective device but it was uncertain if it had been correctly used at the time.

In New Zealand it is mandatory by law for the employer to provide eye

TABLE III

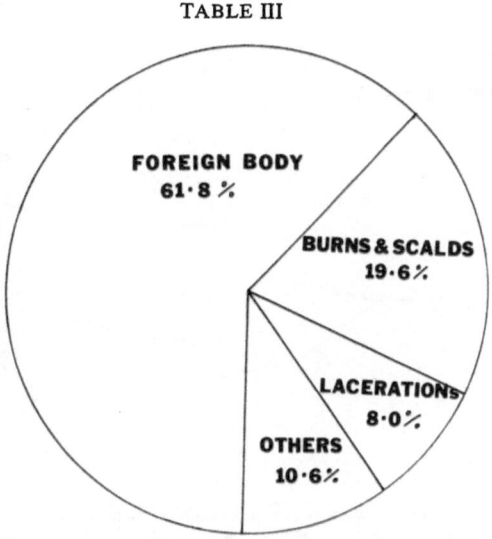

INDUSTRIAL EYE ACCIDENTS

(1961 — 1966)

TABLE IV

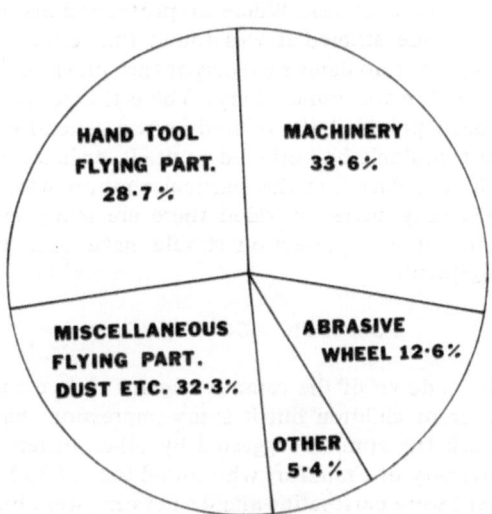

AGENTS CAUSING F.B.

(1966)

TABLE V

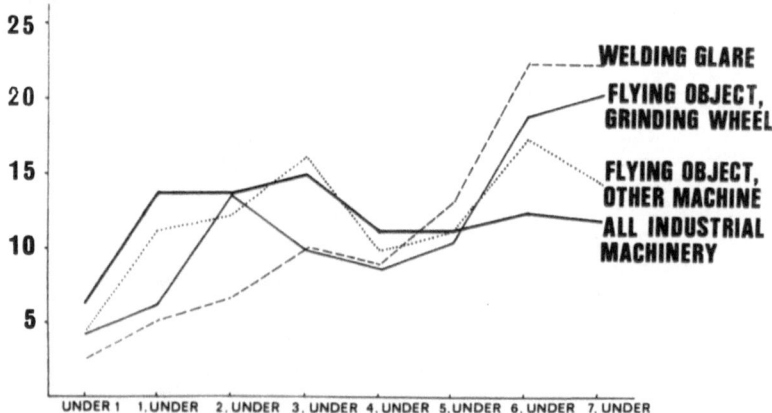

PERCENTAGE OF
0 - 8 HOURS [AVERAGE 1963-1965]

WELDING GLARE

FLYING OBJECT, GRINDING WHEEL

FLYING OBJECT, OTHER MACHINE

ALL INDUSTRIAL MACHINERY

UNDER 1 1. UNDER 2 2. UNDER 3 3. UNDER 4 4. UNDER 5 5. UNDER 6 6. UNDER 7 7. UNDER 8

HOURS ON SHIFT WHEN ACCIDENT OCCURRED — SELECTED MANNERS OF OCCURRENCE WHICH RESULT LARGELY IN EYE INJURIES.

protection for the workers at risk. Where no protection had been provided, in these cases that were studied it was found that either the worker or management thought that no danger existed or that previous experience had indicated that protection was unnecessary. Where the device was not being used and it had been provided the injured person generally thought there was no need or just couldn't be bothered to use it, or had found the device uncomfortable. The conclusion in this particular report was that while eye protection was generally being provided there are many instances where more consideration for eye protection should have been taken both by workers and management.

DOMESTIC ACCIDENTS

I do not have a breakdown of the causative agents of eye accidents occurring in the home or to children but it is my impression that in our series they were very much the same as suggested by other writers e.g. Stark and Hoscht of the University of Frankfurt who found that of 330 eye injuries to children 46 per cent were perforating and 41 per cent were blunt. One third of these were caused by missiles such as shooting or thrown objects, one third by stabbing injury and the other third by thrusts and blows. In our experience the most common missile is probably the stone thrown either by a person or by a rotary lawn mower. Perforating injuries occur from dangerous toys and scissors and bows and arrows. There has been recently a pleasing reduction in the number of injuries from fireworks.

92

DOMESTIC ACCIDENTS

Along with our Department of Public Health the Society for Prevention of Blindness has been active in an advertising campaign to the general public through the national press, radio and television to highlight the dangers of some toys and ask people to be more responsible with fire crackers and sharp instruments. The Society strongly supported a private petition to Parliament requesting it to pass legislation restricting the sale of fireworks. The result of this was two fold: first, much valuable publicity pointing out the dangers to eyesight from fireworks was obtained and secondly it is now illegal to sell fireworks to children for more than one week before Guy Fawkes day. We had hopes to have fireworks banned completely but this has been only a partial success achieved with the banning of the length of the sale of fireworks in the shops to one week in the year.

INDUSTRIAL ACCIDENTS

The National Safety Association is funded through insurance companies compulsorily as part of the premium when an employer insures his workers. It is their responsibility to visit factories and make sure that proper safety devices are provided, to give lectures to management and workers on eye safety. They also sponsor the Wise Owl Club. We are hopeful that there will be some extension of this to domestic accidents now that such accidents are covered by recent legislation in a compulsory national insurance scheme and we hope that the National Safety Association will spread its endeavours into the domestic and farming fields which have not been given as much attention to date as industry.

MOTOR VEHICLE ACCIDENTS

These fortunately have never caused a high percentage of ocular injury but often they cause the most severe ones. There has been a noticeable reduction in ocular as well as general injuries since front seat belts have been worn compulsorily. Legislation has been in force for 6 years making it mandatory for the driver and front seat passenger to wear a diagonal seat belt. I would recommend this legislation to you as far as eye safety is concerned.

SUMMARY

Figures are presented to show the high incidence of ocular injuries in the home. Also the high incidence amongst young children. The causative agents of industrial injuries are reviewed and the fact that workers are more liable to injury when fatigued. Methods of prevention now being undertaken in New Zealand are reviewed.

ACKNOWLEDGEMENTS

I wish to acknowledge help received from DR. CALVIN RING, President of the New Zealand Society for Prevention of Blindness in making facts and figures available to me. The help of Mr. ROSS CLAYTON and the Department of Medical Photography at Waikato Hospital in preparation of the illustrations and my secretary Mrs. K. COWELL in typing the manuscript.

REFERENCES

N.Z. Department of Labour Eye Injuries 1962 to 1966 N.Z. Department Lab. Research Report 1958/5
STARK N. & HOSCHT W. *Med. Klin. Ocular Lesions in Childhood,* 68/9: *274-278* (1973).

PREVENTION OF OCULAR TRAUMA
BY LEGISLATION

KUANG HUI LIM

(Singapore)

Sir STEWART DUKE ELDER in 1972 rightly said: 'trauma is one of the Captains of the Men of Death'.

In discussing the subject of ocular trauma, I wish to address myself to two aspects of prevention about which legislation was recently enacted in Singapore. The Martial Arts Instruction Bill reads partly as follows: 'Organizations which teach martial art, be it a Chinese pugilistic art, or karate or taekwondo or judo or bersilat, aikido, kung fu, jiu jitsu, kendo, in effect equip their members with a potential weapon which, if abused, can have serious consequences for their victims and serious implications for the maintenance of law and order'.

The Bill has more than purely local significance for it emphasizes the grievous consequences of injury that may be seen in countries where martial art is becoming popular, introducing thereby a new dimension in the horrors of ocular trauma. We have seen a number of ocular injuries sustained during practice or in criminal asault cases, as shown in Table I.

Until a few years ago the term martial art was hardly used in Singapore; then came the popularity of Chinese films especially from Hongkong and Taiwan in the late 60s which glorified martial arts and with it the rapid proliferation of martial art organizations in the country. In moving the Bill in Parliament, the Minister said that at the end of 1973 there were 128 organizations in Singapore compared to 32 in 1963, with a number of trainees estimated at between 13,000 and 18,000. The sinister fact was that secret society members and the criminal elements had learnt the art to further their own ends. Apart from criminal assault, the danger of injuries inflicted during training are real, as has been shown, and while on the one hand the Bill was intended to regulate the activities of martial art organizations, on the other, trainees and instructors alike should learn to take added precaution to develop their gaze and reflexes in dodging as the head and face are common targets of blows. Further, spectacle glasses that can shatter should never be worn during practice.

Sir STEWART DUKE ELDER in 1972 said of firecracker injuries: '...practically all such injuries are due to over exuberance or lack of controlling influences and the result of carelessness'. Guy Fawkes may not be familiar in Singapore, but addressing Parliament in moving the Dangerous Fireworks Bill on 2nd June, 1972, the Minister for Home Affairs said: 'The firing of crackers is an ancient Chinese custom, rooted in beliefs no longer credible among the better educated, but, nevertheless, remaining an

TABLE I

Ocular injuries from martial art

Case	Race	Sex	Age	Mechanism	Injury	Visual Result
1	Chinese	M	17	17 Kicked spectacle glasses broke	Corneal laceration	6/9
2	Chinese	F	19	Kicked	Traumatic hyphaema	6/9
3	Chinese	M	26	Kicked	Orbital Fracture, Surgical emphysema & subconjunctival haemorrhage	
4	Chinese	M	30	Fisted (assault)	Orbital blow-out fracture	Persistent diplopia
5	Malay	M	13	Struck by Kris (bersilat)	Eyelid and cheek lacerations	Paralytic squint
6	Chinese	M	27	Kicked	Eyelid laceration subconjunctival haemorrhage	6/6

Key: M = Male
      F = Female

enjoyable way of celebrating Chinese festive occasions, such as the Chinese New Year. The firing of crackers has always presented the problem of fire hazards, which have increased, as the explosive ingredients are improved by modern scientific knowledge. In addition, hazards of physical injuries also have become a problem'. The Minister went on to recount that in Chinese New Year of 1970 there was indiscriminate letting off of fire crackers resulting in 6 deaths, 68 injured and damage to property, then imposed (The Minor Offenses Amendment Act, 1970). The ban was lifted during the Chinese New Year festival but this resulted in 9 persons being injured in 1971 whilst in 1972 members of the public, more bold in their disregard, created more havoc, resulting in 26 persons injured and 2 unarmed policemen brutally attacked. As a result of public outcry, and in view of the numerous breaches of the law and, even more important, the injuries and deaths resulting from the indiscriminate firing of crackers, the Government came to the conclusion that the only practicable solution left was a total ban on the possession of firing or crackers.

Thus, what was once commonplace in our casualty units was totally eradicated and Table II shows the last of firecracker injuries in Singapore in 1972.

TABLE II

Ocular injuries from firecrackers in Singapore

Year	Number Injured	Loss of Sight
1970	40	Monocular blindness (2 cases)
1971	Nil	Nil
1972	5	Nil
1973	Nil	Nil
1974	Nil	Nil

REFERENCES

DUKE ELDER, S. System of Ophthalmology, Vol. XIV, Part I, Injuries, Page V and 19, Kimpton, London, 1972.
Parliamentary Debates Singapore Official Report, 27th March, 1974.

OCULAR ONCHOCERCIASIS: 'AT RISK' PATIENTS AND THEIR TREATMENT

JOHN ANDERSON & HARALD FUGLSANG

(Kumba, S.W. Province, United Cameroon Republic)

INTRODUCTION

Most workers in the field agree that neither of the two drugs currently available for the treatment of onchocerciasis, diethylcarbamazine citrate (DEC) and suramin, are ideal for mass therapy. DEC kills only the microfilariae but not the adult worms. Severe systemic reactions follow its administration and militates against the acceptability of this drug. Furthermore, the administration of the tablets has to be supervised. A two-week course will greatly reduce the number of microfilariae in the skin, yet their concentration soon builds up, and if the vector is present transmission of the disease will be unaffected. Weekly intravenous injections of suramin kill the adult worms as well as some of the microfilariae, but to be effective a course must last four weeks or longer. This drug has proved too toxic for mass administration. Nodulectomy campaigns performed twice a year in Guatemala have not altered the prevalence of onchocerciasis, though they may have reduced the blindness rates.

The best approach in the fight against onchocerciasis appears to be vector control. However, in areas where such control is possible, and even in progress, there remain many candidates for blindness among the heavily infected. It would therefore seem essential to find these 'at risk' patients and to give them the best available treatment.

MATERIALS AND METHODS

The following account is based on work carried out in a heavily infected savanna focus in northern Cameroon during the past four years.

In 1971 and 1972, total populations aged five years and over were surveyed in four villages (a, b, c, and d) at distances of 2, 3, 7, and 25 kilometers, respectively, from the nearest perennial Simulium breeding site. Village d was close to a stream with seasonal breeding. Weighed skin snips were taken at the left shoulder and buttock, and the number of microfilariae per mg of skin (mf/mg) was calculated. The number and location of palpable nodules were recorded. Central vision was tested by means of an illiterate E-chart. The anterior segments of the eyes were examined with a Haag-Streit 900 slit lamp, and the posterior segments with a direct ophthalmoscope or an indirect binocular model. The number of microfilariae seen in the cornea, anterior chamber, and vitreous was recorded.

99

In 1973, when the full confidence of the people had been obtained, 100 patients with microfilariae in the eye were selected for treatment from these villages, together with an additional 200 patients who came spontaneously with eye symptoms from nearby villages.

These 300 selected cases were then treated with either DEC or suramin, or by nodulectomy, alone or in different combinations. Twenty patients who received placebo injections served as controls. The DEC course consisted of 25 mg on day 1, 25 mg morning and evening on day 2, 50 mg morning and evening on day 3, and then an additional 50 mg daily for a total dose of 200 mg morning and evening, continued for 5-7 days. In some patients this was followed by suppressive DEC, i.e., a weekly dose of 200 mg. The suramin course consisted of weekly injections of 1 g — or less according to weight — for 4-6 weeks.

Before treatment the patients were examined and two additional quantitative skin snips were taken from the outer canthus of the eye and the lower calf, respectively. The patients were followed closely during and following treatment. The study is still in progress.

RESULTS AND DISCUSSION

Only results bearing on risk and treatment will be discussed.

Risk Factors

1. Community Risk Factors.

The distances of the four villages from the nearest perennial Simulium breeding site were different, but the prevalence figures for onchocerciasis were almost the same, 93.8 percent, 98.0 percent, 95.0 percent, and 88.8 percent at villages a, b, c, and d, respectively. However, the corresponding blindness rates in people of 20 years of age and over were 13.6, 14.4, 4.0, and 0 percent, while for males of 20 years and over, they were 21.0, 20.6, 6.2, and 0 percent.

The mean density of mf/mg skin and the number of microfilariae in the eye correspond closely to the blindness rates in each of these villages. The intensity of infection was thus closely related to the proximity of the village to the perennial Simulium breeding site, and it is the intensity rather than the prevalence of infection which determines the severity of ocular onchocerciasis in a community.

2. Individual Risk Factors.

The higher blindness rates found in males than in females may be explained by hormonal differences, since the exposure to Simulium bites in the village and in the fields was probably similar for both sexes. It is possible, however, that the men and boys spent more time fishing and hunting near the rivers. A high proportion of the patients who presented themselves with ocular onchocerciasis gave a history of camping for some months close to a river, either for farming, fishing, or hunting. In southern Sudan, we came across a

100

river ferry which was manned by three completely blind and one partially blind ferrymen. However, it is difficult to separate the relative roles of hormonal and occupational factors in the development of severe lesions in onchocerciasis.

Of the 200 patients – 157 males and 43 females – who came because of eye symptoms, 70 (35 percent) were under 20 years of age. This points to the early onset of eye changes in onchocerciasis.

3. Risk Symptoms and Signs.

It was impossible to obtain reliable histories of the onset of symptoms, but watering and photophobia were often present at some stage. These symptoms can be a warning of important ocular changes in onchocerciasis, but they can also be due to trachoma and less important eye conditions. In many lesions of the posterior segment of the eye, night blindness was an early presenting symptom.

Impairment of vision was common, but in 48 patients (24 percent) there was good central vision – 6/9 or better in either eye – and they might therefore have passed a superficial vision test. However, though visual fields were not tested routinely, in 12 of these 48 patients they were obviously grossly restricted. Such restriction is undoubtedly an important early sign in lesions of the optic nerve in onchocerciasis.

In 93 percent microfilariae were seen in the cornea, usually in appreciable numbers – 20 or more. In 76 percent they were present in the anterior chamber, and in 19 percent in the vitreous. In 5 percent, 10 percent and 20 percent, respectively, microfilariae would not be seen in the cornea, anterior chamber, and vitreous because of opacities. Although these prevalence figures are all higher than in a total population in a highly endemic area, the most striking feature was the much higher number of microfilariae seen per eye in these patients.

In Africa comparatively little importance has been attached to the head nodule in onchocerciasis. It is interesting to note therefore that a palpable nodule was present on the head in 26.5 percent of the 200 patients. In the total village populations in the same area, head nodules were only palpated in about 1 percent. Patients with head nodules showed a higher average microfilarial concentration in the skin at the outer canthus (52 mf/mg) than those without head nodules (37 mf/mg). However, it is possible that impalpable head nodules were present in many patients in this latter group, since 25 percent of them showed more than 50 mf/mg in the skin at the outer canthus. Although the patients with head nodules also had higher concentrations of microfilariae at the buttock than those without head nodules, it is our opinion that a quantitative snip taken at the outer canthus is a better indicator than a buttock or any other snip of possible danger to the eye.

In summary, the candidates for blindness due to onchocerciasis were particularly the males in villages close to a perennial Simulium breeding site. They might be recognized before the onset of irreversible visual impairment by the presence of a head nodule, or by finding many microfilariae in the cornea, anterior chamber, or in the skin around the eye. The symptoms of watering, photophobia, and night blindness should not be ignored.

Treatment

In the control group there were no marked changes in the numbers of microfilariae seen in the eye. The visual acuity was mainly unchanged, but two patients required treatment because they developed iritis during the year of follow-up. Two other patients died of causes thought to be unrelated to onchocerciasis.

Diethylcarbamazine.

The immediate general reactions were so severe that only a small percentage would have continued after the first day without a considerable amount of persuasion and encouragement. However, we have also worked in a severe focus in northern Nigeria, and there the people were so keen on DEC treatment that they queued up for it, and many refused to take aspirin with it since they wanted to experience the full effect of the drug. A medical geographer had been working on onchocerciasis in that area for a year, and it is likely that he had created a demand for treatment.

In this Cameroon focus, five out of fifteen patients collapsed during the first four days of DEC treatment. Their initial dose was 50 mg. Patients treated were always heavily parasitized and we subsequently gave routine steroid coverage during the two days before treatment and continued it during the first five to six days of treatment. In this way it was possible to control the side effects to some extent. The following description therefore is of this combined treatment.

Even under steroid cover groin lymphadenopathy was often so severe as to make walking almost impossible. Twice daily doses of 200 mg DEC often caused vertigo, and it is doubtful whether it is advisable or necessary to increase the dose to that level.

After a period of watering and redness, the eyes usually settled within a day or two. The microfilariae in the cornea died, and those in the anterior chamber were reduced in numbers. The drug had a remarkably beneficial effect on corneal symptomatology, and the sudden death of hundreds of larvae in the cornea did not lead to an increase in keratitis. Likewise in the anterior chamber there was in general no increase in signs of anterior uveitis during DEC therapy.

At the follow-up examination after a year, the microfilariae in the cornea and in the anterior chamber were almost at their pretreatment levels. Visual acuity was not significantly altered by DEC treatment, and improvements in signs and symptoms were only temporary.

Suppressive diethylcarbamazine.

Of the 40 patients who started suppressive DEC, less than half followed it regularly, and most of those had to be persuaded to do so. The main objection was itching after each weekly dose. A lightly infected man in whom the initial DEC course had eliminated almost all microfilariae from his skin did not experience this itching. It is therefore possible that suppressive DEC would be more acceptable if the initial course was three to four weeks long to eliminate almost all the microfilariae.

Only ten patients in this group have been followed for a year, but it appeared that the numbers of microfilariae present both in the cornea and anterior chamber were reduced. Particularly striking were some corneas in which the microfilariae, previously counted in hundreds, were kept at very small numbers. In two cases with very severe iritis, the anterior chambers became much quieter following DEC therapy and remained so on the suppressive regime.

Suramin.

On the whole the first four injections were well accepted. Only one patient out of the first hundred treated refused to attend after the first injection, while a further ten had to be persuaded to complete the course. Lack of immediate improvement in both symptoms and visual acuity, and sometimes an aggravation of symptoms, had an adverse effect on the acceptance of the injections.

Of the first one hundred patients, many did not complete the course because of severe general reactions such as stomatitis, dermatitis, and general malaise. As many as 50 percent were so prostrated shortly after completing the course that for a week or more they were unable to carry out even light work. In two patients, both of whom had received four injections, the prostration continued and led to death three to four months later. One was a boy of 15, and the other a middle-aged woman. In one other patient the liver was slightly enlarged before treatment. He felt so prostrated after his second injection that no more were given. He improved slightly but later died in a state of coma one month after the second injection. One young man developed exfoliative dermanitis a week after the fifth injection. He was very ill but gradually recovered on corticosteroid therapy.

After the third or fourth injection, pronounced reactions often developed around the microfilariae in the cornea. Where stromal keratitis was present, it was usually aggravated. At about the same time 25 percent developed signs of mild uveal irration in the form of a fine flare and cells in the anterior chamber. A further 13 percent developed more serious signs of anterior uveitis with heavy flare and fresh keratic precipitates, and three other patients developed anterior uveitis of sufficient severity to cause posterior synechiae. Suramin treatment was discontinued in three cases because of the onset of iritis. These complications were not directly correlated with the number of microfilariae seen in the anterior chambers pre-treatment, nor with the presence or absence of signs of previous attacks of iritis.

The follow-up at a year after treatment showed a tremendous reduction in the prevalence of microfilariae in the cornea ranging from 91 percent to 6 percent. When still present they were seen only in very small numbers, never more than 5 per cornea. At the same follow-up microfilariae were seen in the anterior chamber in 14 percent of cases, compared with 80 percent pre-treatment, and the 'suramin-induced' iritis had largely disappeared. Eyes which had shown signs of active keratitis or anterior uveitis pre-treatment were generally quieter, but there were no marked changed in lesions of the posterior segment.

There was no real change in visual acuity following treatment in the majority of patients.

Among 25 patients in whom the number of microfilariae had been greatly reduced by a two-week course of DEC prior to sumarin administration, signs of mild uveal irration developed in only two, and of more severe irration in one. Anterior uveitis complications were fewer when the microlarial load had been reduced before suramin treatment. This was true also of dermatitis and general malaise.

Nodulectomy.

This procedure was quite popular in our area. Only ten patients have been followed for a year after removal of all palpable nodules. There were no significant changes in the number of microfilariae seen in the cornea and anterior chamber, but the number in the skin was reduced to 63 percent of its pre-treatment level.

In patients in whom the eyes and skin are heavily parasitized, nodulectomy alone should probably not be expected to produce much benefit since many impalpable nodules are likely to be present. However, nodules on the head undoubtedly constitute an added hazard to the eye, and their removal is always advisable.

SUMMARY AND CONCLUSIONS

In view of the severity of the reactions caused by both DEC and suramin, neither drug is suitable for mass treatment. However, these reactions can be controlled to some extent, and effective elimination of the parasite is possible. Such elimination can prevent or halt the further development of sclerosing keratitis and anterior uveitis, which are the two most important causes of blindness due to onchocerciasis in the savanna. Its effect on the posterior segment of the eye is still not clear.

As the optimum treatment we recommend a course of DEC lasting 15-20 days under initial steroid cover in order to 'quieten' the eyes and to kill a large proportion of the microfilariae and thus dampen subsequent general and ocular reactions; followed by weekly injections of suramin to a total dose of about 100 mg/kg. Ideally all nodules, and particularly those on the head, should be removed.

Such a regime could be carried out effectively by mobile teams in villages with a high intensity of infection where there may be 5 percent or more 'at risk' patients. An ophthalmologist should be in charge, but even so the selection of patients in need of treatment is not always easy. Some eyes for instance seem to reach an equilibrium with their parasite, so that they are not in particular need of treatment.

We suggest that specially trained paramedical staff might use the following criteria as a basis for the preliminary selection of 'at risk' patients, to be submitted to a medical officer as possible cases for treatment:

1. more than 50 microfilariae in the cornea
2. more than 20 microfilariae in the anterior chamber
3. more than 25 mf/mg skin at the outer canthus
4. the presence of a head nodule
5. the onset of night blindness

It is needless to point out that the success of such a program would depend entirely on the time and care taken in explaining its purpose to the villagers, and on the dedication of the staff.

PROBLEMS IN THE TREATMENT OF ONCHOCERCIASIS

M.M.O. BEIRAM

(Khartoum, Sudan)

Onchocerciasis in the Sudan is characterized by dermal lesions, nodule formations and ocular complications. It has been noted that the pattern and distribution of these lesions differs from one endemic area to another. Factors that may explain these disparities include nutrition, local immunity, intensity and duration of infection and probably the habits of the vector.

GEOGRAPHICAL DESCRIPTION

The Northern province is an almost rainless desert region which suffers extremes of hot dry weather in summer and cold dry weather in winter. The population, predominantly Arabs and Muslims, occupy cultivated areas separated by sparsely populated rocky and sandy spaces. The disease is found in the area extending between the 4th and 5th cataracts where the river is rocky and dotted with a number of islands.

The province of Bahr El Ghazal is a clssical savannah area crossed by a large number of annual and perennial rivers. It is inhabited by negroid people. The immense distances involved and the rough nature of the country with its many waterways pose considerable problems in the treatment of the human reservoir or the vector.

CLINICAL FEATURES

Abu Hamed Focus

An outstanding feature at this focus is the low microfilaria load found in skin biopsies. Only 35 microfilariae were detected out of 62 snips examined. This constitutes an overall 0.27 mf. per mgm. of skin.

The prevalence rate of the disease varied between 8.0% on parasitological diagnosis to 16.0% on clinical assessment. The frequency of ocular complications was 5.5 to 6.9%. One of the main symptoms is itching. Dermatological changes significantly linked to onchocerciasis are:
1. Papules, macules or nodules that appear during the early stage of the disease; thickening and dark discoloration of the skin and depigmentation that classically affects the tibial areas.
2. Dermatological changes involved the lower limbs, the pelvic area, the chest, the neck and rarely the upper limbs. They never involved the whole body.

3. Nodules were detected in 6.9% of the cases.

In 1973, BEIRAM studied onchocercal ocular complications in this region. He found 5.7% bilateral blindness. Chronic iritis, punctate keratitis and choroidoretinitis were the main causes. Deformities of the pupil optic atrophy did not occur.

Bahr El Ghazal Focus

In a quantitative study at Wau town, 1683 microfilariae were detected in 205 snips, an overall 3.3 mf per mg. skin. This is almost twelve times the concentration found at Abu Hamed. As many as 100-200 mf. could be counted in some of the snips during repeated examinations. BEIRAM in 1973 found that the concentration of mf. skin biopsies was similar to records from other savannah areas in Africa. Females in his series showed significantly lower loads than males in a ratio of 0.4 to 4.7 mf. per mgm.

Onchocerciasis is the major cause of blindness in this province. Bilateral blindness was diagnosed in 4.9% and unilateral in 2.7%. With advancing age blindness increased, so that at 50 years of age almost 20.0% of the population was blind. BEIRAM in 1973 found anterior segment lesions twice as often as posterior segment lesions. Eye lesions included sclerosing and punctate keratitis, superficial corneal opacities and iridocyclitis with synechiae. The commonest posterior segment involvements were choroidosclerosis, pigment migration and optic atrophy.

In areas with a high incidence of bilateral blindness for economic, sociological and humanitarian reasons vector control and chemotherapy should be tried. The terrain, the mixed races and languages, the flooding of rivers and proximal marsh land during the rains as well as the varying ways of life in the South make treatment a formidable problem.

Chemotherapy is unpopular in both the North and the South. Distances are immense. Terrain and communications make travel difficult. Unless treatment is carried out by a global authority such as the World Health Organization using airplanes, it is difficult to envisage success.

IMMUNOLOGICAL CONCEPTIONS OF THE TREATMENT AND PREVENTION OF ONCHOCERCIASIS

M. MOJON

(Lyon, France)

The first step in approaching this problem is to consider the possibilities of preventive vaccination against onchocerciasis.

This affection in fact, is one of the major preoccupations of large international organizations such as the W.H.O. and the governments of countries in which it is endemic. It appears difficult to eradicate onchocerciasis by taking action against the vectors only: pilot experiments carried out have not always given satisfactory results up till now. The mirofilaricide drugs at present available, which are a necessary complement to this action, are not entirely harmless and are difficult to handle in mass treatment.

It may be asked whether vaccination would not be a useful adjuvant in the campaign against onchocerciasis, a disease whose social and economic effects are widely recognized — whole populations condemned to inactivity because of ocular complications, and fertile regions deserted.

The first part of this article deals with veterinary research and its results, together with work in progress with a view to its application in human medicine.

Consideration will then be given to the question of vaccination against onchocerciasis and the problems involved in its realization.

In conclusion we shall define the preliminary studies that seem to us necessary before this hypothetic vaccine can be produced, particularly the neccessity of establishing with certitude the pathogenic mechanism of the ocular lesions and the contribution that a study of healthy populations living in endemic areas could provide.

I. WORK ALREADY ACCOMPLISHED

Research into active immunization against certain parasites has been intensified during the last twenty years, particularly with regard to helminths. Veterinary medicine has greatly benefited from the results. Without going into details of all these works, several will be summarized in an attempt to emphasize what we consider important points for possible application to onchocerciasis: methods of preparing vaccines, route of administration and preservation of vaccines.

Three types of vaccine can be defined:

a) Vaccinating substances prepared from exo-antigens

These substances are prepared from the excretion-secretion products of infesting larvae.

TALIAFERRO had already discovered the immunogenic value of metabolic products of Ascaris larvae in 1943, followed by SPRENT et al. in 1949. SOULSBY (1957 - 1958) showed that production of immunogenic antigens is perceptible mainly at the L2 → L3 sloughing season, and this author observed that L3 larvae are particularly affected by protective antobodies. The immunogenic power of exo-antigens was also used for attempts to immunize against *Trichinella spiralis Nippostrongylus muris*, etc.

More recently WONG, FREDERICKS & RAMACHANDRAN (1969) used exo-antigens of *Brugia malayi* for experimental vaccination of Rhesus monkeys against lymphatic filariasis. For this purpose the authors incubated L3 larvae of *B. malayi* for one hour at $37°C$ in 1.25 ml sterile KREBS-RINGER solution. The animals were injected subcutaneously with 1 ml of the supernatant fluid in the injections at 15 days' interval. This 'vaccination' was followed by inoculation with 100 live L3 larvae. The immunization thus obtained did not prevent the infection from developing, but the intensity and duration of microfilaremia were less, than in control animals.

b) Vaccinating substances obtained by incubating infesting larvae in hyperimmune serum

Investigators used this method very early. The first works cited by WONG et al. are those of MAUS in 1940, which were continued by OLIVIER-GONZALES, SSCHWABE, etc. In immunization trials of Rhesus monkeys against *B. malayi* WONG et al. left L3 larvae in contact with 1 ml of hyperimmune serum for one hour at $37°C$. This serum was taken from monkeys infested with 20 successive doses of 20 live infesting larvae, microfilaremia having been negative in these animals for one year. These authors, in fact, criticize this method themselves, since application in immunofluorescence in the search for antibodies showed that the antibodies found in the hyperimmune serum were directed against microfilariae and not against infesting larvae. Moreover, the results of this immunization are entirely superposable on those obtained with exo-antigens (WONG et al. 1969).

Vaccinating substances prepared with radiated L3 larvae

It is in this field that the most numerous experimentations have taken place with the most convincing results.

Infesting larvae were radiated either with X-rays or with γ rays. Work of this kind has been carried out with many types of helminths: *Ascaris, Haemonchys contortus, Trichostrongylus colubris, Dictyocaulus viviparus, Dictyocaulus filaria, Ancylostoma canimum, Uncinaria stenocephala.*

The greatest progress in this field is due to JARRETT and his team. The first experimentations concerned *D. viviparus* responsible for parasitic bronchitis in bovines. The results may be summarized as follows: live L3 larvae were radiated with 40.000 r. for 8 hours, then administered by mouth to animals aged 2-3 months at a dose of about 1.000 larvae per animal.

The vaccinal dose was repeated 4 weeks later. Twenty days after the second dose of vaccine the calves were put out to pasture in an infested area.

Unlike the control group, the vaccinated animals showed no signs of parasitic bronchitis and weight gain was normal. These experiments in the field confirm the results obtained by the authors in the laboratory (JARRETT et al., 1959, 1960, 1961). POYNTER (1963), working on the same subject, considered that the interval between the two doses of vaccine could be reduced to 15 days. TOMANEK also obtained goods results in Chechoslovakia by subcutaneous injection of radiated larvae..

The same type of experiments have since been attempted with radiated L3 larvae of *D. filaria* administered to ovines. JOVANOVIC found a "DIFIL" vaccine prepared in Yugoslovakia satisfactory, but KASSAY et al. In Irak contested the value of this vaccine, as they obtained much better protection of ovines with non-radiated L3 larvae. However, these authors reported that the second vaccinal dose had expired 12 days before they used it.

MILLER effectively protected young dogs against *A. canium* by subcutaneous injection of a dose of radiated L3 larvae at 2 week's interval. This author went on to state that the immunity thus conferred enabled puppies to resist both experimental reinfestation by non-radiated larvae at a normally lethal dose and also natural reinfestation when the animals were placed in a highly infested area. Ideal protection is obtained when vaccination is carried out at the age of 2 or 3 months, but the author also obtained immunity – less reliable, it is true – when vaccination was performed on dogs aged 3 days.

Work by DOW et al. on *U. stenocephale* shows that radiation of L3 larvae by 20,000 and 40,000 r. inhibits the evolution of these parasitic forms and prevents their transformation into adult worms, while preserving their immunogenic properties. However, these properties are best preserved by radiation at doses of 20,000 r., and the best resistance is obtained by administering 1,000 radiated larvae at 4 weeks' interval.

With regard to work carried out on *B. malayi* several doses of X-rays were experimented. The authors consider the most effective to be 20,000 r. The bumber of larvae per vaccinal dose is 200 (the authors tried vaccines containing 100, 200 and 400 larvae, respectively radiated at 10,000, 20,000 and 40,000 r.). Under these conditions, no infection was found in any of the treated Rhesus monkeys after test inoculation with non-attenuated live larvae. The protection was maintained for more than 10 months, but two perfectly developed filariae (one male and one female) were found in a monkey who had never suffered from microfilaremia (WONG et al., 1969)

Other experiments were performed both on helminthiasis and protozoosis. In the latter category we refer particularly to attempts to perfect a vaccine against malaria.

In this connection we would like to point out the following: – the works of CORADETTI, who irradiated either the sporozoites or erythrocytal forms of the parasite, and who considered that protection, which was only partial, was obtained only against the parasitic stages used in the vaccinating substances. The advantage of this research from the author's point of view was to afford better protection against pernicious attacks on children and newly arrived subjects, rather than totally immunizing them against malaria (oral communication).

— the works of Mrs. NUSSENZWIEG, whose studies concerned the immunogenic of different plasmodial stages taking place in the vector, and who showed that only sporozoites accumulated in the salivary glands of mosquitoes are immunogenic, and the longer they remain in the glands the greater their immunogenic power. This author also attempted to increase the vaccinating power of sporozoites by using stimulants of cellular immunity of bacterial type administered by repeated intra-dermo reaction. For this purpose she used both complete and incomplete Freud adjuvant, whooping cough bacillus, and aims at. continuing her work with *Corynebacterium parvum* (oral communication.)

Radiation was performed by X-rays in all cases referred to above, but many authors used γ rays emitted by 60 Co. — for example, FETENAU et al. for attenuating larvae of *Syngamus trachea*, BITAKARAMIRE for metacercariae of *Fasciola gigantiea*, PURNELL et al. and PHILLIPS for attenuating *Babesia major* and *Babesia rodhaini* respectively, DUXBURY and SADUN for *Trypanosoma rhodesiense*.

Before concluding this part of the article devoted to methods of preparing vaccinating substances, reference should be made to the works of CORNWELL & JONES (1970) who submitted larvae of *N. brasiliensis* and *D. viviparus* to the action of a cytotoxic agent, triethylene melamine, and attenuated them to a point at which their immunizing role proved equal to that of radiated larvae. The experiments gave the same results whether carried out in the laboratory or the field.

To demonstrate the merits of research aimed at perfecting a vaccine against onchocerciasis, we have rapidly reviewed the work already carried out in veterinary medicine in order to emphasize the very positive results obtained. It would have been long and wearisome to reiterate the experimental methods each time, so we shall summarize them in a few points, always with the idea of their application to onchocerciasis.

1. To obtain valid vaccinating substances, infesting larvae must be used at the third stage.

2. Radiation seems the best method at present available for attenuating infesting larvae without at the same time destroying their immunogenic power.

3. Type of radiation: X-rays and γ rays: this is important only with regard to dose of radiation. Although the results are contradictory, it appears that an equivalent dose, X-rays generally provide better attenuation than γ rays. However, according to FITZPATRICK & MULLIGAN 1967 this difference would disappear if instead of considering the number of adult worms found in animals used in the experiment, the ratio of adult females to adult males were taken into account. The percentage of males reaching adult stage seems to decrease considerably under the effect of radiation.

4. Conditions of radiation should be exactly defined as regards duration,

112

temperature and oxygenation of the medium in which the larvae develop. There is marked decrease in radiosensivity of larvae when the temperature is increased, particularly between 20° C and 30° C. This phenomenon is probably connected with more rapid reduction of oxygen in the medium, indicating increased metabolic activity of the larvae under the effect of heat.

5. The success obtained by CORNWELL & JONES, using a cytotoxic agent to attenuate infesting larvae merits attention.

6. The number of larvae contained in each vaccinal dose is very variable from one experiment to another: 200 for the Rhesus monkey, 1,000 for calves, etc. At first sight it seems in proportion to the weight of the animals.

7. The route of administration of the 'vaccines' is generally that naturally adopted by the parasites, although this seems to have only relative importance is TOMANEK's results are considered.

8. The age at which the subjects are vaccinated plays an important role in all the works cited, with the exception of that of MILLER on puppies. All authors generally admit that precocious vaccination when the defence systems are still immature carries the risk of hampering later acquisition of immunity, sometimes completely.

9. Furthermore, it would be desirable of define:

- The duration of validity of vaccines (therein perhaps lies the advantage of cytotoxic agents)
- preservation temperature (an important problem in the case of onchocerciasis)
- the duration of the protection
- finally, the immunization time-table.

II. POSSIBLE PROJECTS OF ACTIVE IMMUNIZATION AGAINST ONCHOCERCIASIS

The main interest of protection against onchocerciasis is because of the handicapping character of the affection, whose ocular complications can paralyze a high percentage of the population during its period of economic activity.

a) Protection against infesting larvae

It may be stated here and now that the use of radiated larvae of the third stage has some chance of being effective against the development of healthy larvae inoculated during the vector-receptor contact.

A certain number of difficulties are encountered in perfecting a vaccinating suspension against onchocerciasis, the most important of which is obtaining the larvae.

To do so, an experimental laboratory cycle must be contemplated, which means that:

1. an animal receptive to *Onchocerca volvulus* must be found, in which development of the parasite would be comparable to that in man. DUKE's works on inoculation of *O. volvulus* in chimpanzees prove that at least one animal species is sensitive to this filaria. It would obviously be desirable to find an animal species sensitive to *O. volvulus* which would be easier to

manage in the laboratory and less costly to acquire than chimpanzees.

2. Simulia bred must be capable of ensuring transmission and perpetuity of the affection, at the same time providing the number of larvae necessary to produce the vaccines.

The number of infesting Simulium larvae is known to be very low, and highly developed breeding of vectors would be necessary.

3. alternatively, an axenic culture of helminths must be attempted. Chick chorio-allantois was used for the culture of monoxenous and heteroxenous Trematoda, and it was thus possible to develop metacercariae to the adult stage. FRIED obtained viable eggs in this way from adult *Clinostorum marginatum* derived from decysted metacercariae cultivated in this type of medium (1970).

Other types of media were used for these cultures, composed principally of embryonal extracts or extracts of organs, particularly liver, with the addition of serum, salts and vitamins, and placed in atmosphere with a defined percentage of nitrogen, carbon dioxide and oxygen.

FIORAVANTI kept adult *Hymenolepis diminuta* aged 6 days in diphasic medium and observed increase in weight and the number of proglottides of the worms during the 120-hour experiment (1970).

On the other hand, BERTZEN used axenic culture to obtain 20 successive generations of *Hymenolepis nana* (1970).

These examples are given with the sole aim of eventual application to culture of *O. volvulus* so as to obtain infesting larvae of the third stage.

In any case, once the cycle is obtained, another difficulty arises: how should the larvae be attenuated?

Radiation could be used on the flies, who would then suck the blood of the subjects to be vaccinated. Despite the technical difficulties that can readily be understood, it would seem easier to recuperate infesting larvae by dissecting the salivary glands of infested Simulia or from axenic cultures, and then radiate them.

Finally, it would also be useful to carry out research on the adjuvants of immunity at the same time. Although the mechanism of immunitary defence in parasitoses is not completely clear, it is generally admitted that cellular immunity takes an active part. It is therefore necessary to envisage stimulation of this means of defence by repeated intra-dermo-reactions with bacterial agents. Repeated administration of B.C.G. has been proposed for this purpose in the treatment of acute leukemia. Research is in progress on the possible role of the whooping cough bacillus, *Corynebacterium parvum* and should be applied in attempts at active immunization against onchocerciasis.

b) Protection against microfilaria in the eye

There are two theories as to the pathogenesis of ocular lesions. - RODGER believes that ocular lesions are provoked by toxins released during death of the microfilaria. The phenomenon observed during the SCHICK reaction seems to be reproduced by experimental inoculation of dead microfilaria in the eye of healthy subjects, onchocercal subjects prior to ocular invasion by microfilaria and onchocercal subjects suffering from ocular invasion but without lesions (RODGER, 1960).

Under these conditions, efforts should be directed towards isolating this toxin in order to manufacture an anatoxin. In 1958 LAGRAULET announced that he was continuing his work on isolating this toxin begun two years previously, and was carrying out a physiopathological study.

However, even if an anatoxin was obtained, it might still be wondered to what extent its injection would produce a circulating antitoxin that would protect the eye.
- Many other authors consider that the action of microfilaria in the eye is allergic.

It is obvious, in fact, that it is often difficult to distinguish between toxic and allergic elements, particularly in helminthology. It would, however, be necessary to reach agreement on this point. An allergic pathogenic mechanism, in fact, should lead to greater prudence in administering a vaccine which might exceed its purpose and create a state of harmful reactional hypersensitivity in the eye.

III. PRELIMINARY STUDIES

Differences of opinion on the mechanism of the lesions that represent the severity of onchocerciasis lead us to believe that certain points should be cleared up before beginning work on vaccination.
They are twofold:
- a precise definition of the pathogenic mechanism of ocular lesions
- a study of healthy subjects living in endemic areas.

a) Pathogenic mechanism

Experimental inoculation of live and killed microfilaria in rabbit eye, together with a detailed pathological study have confirmed RODGERS's opinion of the toxic mechanism of ocular lesions (1960). NEUMANN experimented on the chimpanzee eye and also considered that the lesions were connected with the death and disintegration of microfilaria (NEUMANN et al., 1964) He did not go further in his pathogenic explanation.

DUKE who also took the rabbit as an experimental animal, tried to prove the existence of a difference in virulence between the savanna and forest strains of O. volvulus. Unlike RODGER, he concluded that ocular lesions were provoked by live microfilaria. The author admitted that a few microfilaria could have died before being inoculated, but was nevertheless in favour of a pathogenic mechanism of allergic origin whose sequence he explained from his point of view (DUKE & ANDERSON, 1971; Garner, DUKE & ANDERSON, 1973).
In the face of such differences of opinion, it seems necessary for experiments of this type to be repeated with uniform experimental procedures. Indeed, if RODGER's viewpoint were confirmed, it would be very important to perform comparable works to those of LAGRAULET in order to isolate a toxin (1958). However, a last remark should be made, namely that RODGER's results might be explained not by the action of a toxin, but by that of an enzyme released by the death of microfilaria, causing the

formation of an anti-enzyme in the eye, which would provoke a reaction similar to that of SCHICK.

b) Studies of healthy populations

Until now the study of onchocerciasis has been mainly carried out on onchocercal subjects, although no explanation has yet been found for the mechanisms of the lesions. The problem could be taken in reverse order, investigating the reason why healthy populations living in endemic areas resist infestation. The interaction of nutritional factors has been envisaged. Several authors have examined the influence of hypovitaminose A in the installation of ocular lesions, and have effectively found this vitamin deficiency in subjects with onchocerciasis. However, these studies are incomplete and should also be extended to healthy subjects. Other deficiencies might also be responsible, such as hypovitaminosis B, etc.

The different responses of subjects submitted to the same risks of infestation may depend on dissimilar immunity connected with particular factors. The present-day possibility of easy quantity determination of the different immunoglobulins and precise exploration of cellular and humoral immunity responses might find application in a comparative study of populations suffering from onchocerciasis and those remaining unaffected.

It would also be useful to investigate whether interference between different helminths, even antigenically distant, plays a part in protecting some subjects from onchocerciasis in those countries where polyparasitism flourishes.

All things considered, the severity of the ocular complications of onchocerciasis appears a sufficient reason for perfecting a vaccine for the active immunization of populations exposed to bites by infested Simulia. However, this work, whose difficulty can easily be imagined, cannot in our opinion be undertaken until the pathogenic mechanism of ocular lesions is established with certainty. For this purpose we consider that in addition to experimental studies carried out on the same basis by teams holding different theories, the natural of acquired resistance factors of healthy subjects living in endemic areas must be elucidated.

All the same, a vaccine of this kind should not be considered a panacea. It can only be a complement to the other two methods of eradicating the disease, that is, destruction of vectors and treatment of affected subjects.

PATHOGENESIS OF CENTRAL
RETINAL VEIN OCCLUSION

SOHAN SINGH HAYREH

(Iowa City, Iowa)

The subject of the pathogenesis of so-called central retinal vein occlusion has been of great controversy for nearly a century since its first description by MICHEL in 1878. A proper understanding of this subject is important for the better management of this common disorder associated with marked visual disturbances. I have reviewed and discussed this subject in detail elsewhere, based on my experimental (1965) and clinical (1971) findings. Further clinical studies have confirmed my previous views.

My experimental studies (1965) in rhesus monkeys showed that:

1. Occlusion of the central retinal vein at its site of exit from the optic nerve was associated with engorged and turgid retinal veins only, and with no other findings attributed to so-called central retinal vein occlusion in patients.

2. Simultaneous occlusion of the central retinal vein and artery at their site of exit and entry respectively from the optic nerve produced the classical clinical picture usually associated with so-called central retinal vein occlusion in patients, i.e., extensive retinal hemorrhages, retinal edema, and marked retinal damage, etc.

From these findings I concluded that retinal arterial ischemia is an important factor in the production of the clinical picture of so-called central retinal vein occlusion.

Further clinical and fluorescein fundus angiographic studies (1971) on the patients with central retinal vascular occlusion confirmed the above conclusions.

Based on these studies, I recommend the following terminology to describe the various types of central retinal vascular occlusions:

1. *Ischemic retinopathy* - due to central retinal artery occlusion.

2. *Venous stasis retinopathy* - due to central retinal vein occlusion behind the lamina cribrosa (not to be confused with an entity described under the same name by KEARNS et al. (1963).

3. *Hemorrhagic retinopathy* - due to central retinal vein occlusion associated with central retinal arterial occlusion.

Fluorescein fundus angiography has revealed that in ischemic retinopathy, the retinal arterial circulation re-establishes itself within a few hours or days, (HAYREH 1971, ...) and in some cases ischemic retinopathy may be due to only a partial occlusion of the central retinal artery. In venous stasis retinopathy the angiography shows venous stasis, engorged capillaries,

117

some microaneurysms and retino-ciliary veins on the optic disc (helping to drain the blood from the retinal veins into the chloroidal veins) (Fig. 1). In

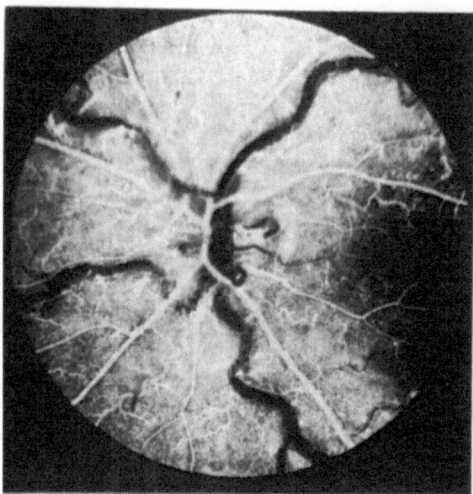

Fig. 1. Fluorescein fundus angiogram during retinal arterial phase in a patient with venous stasis retinopathy.

hemorrhagic retinopathy, on the other hand, there is a classical angiographic appearance showing areas of capillary obliteration, arteriovenous shunts, neovascularization, microaneurysms and retino-ciliary veins (Fig. 2),

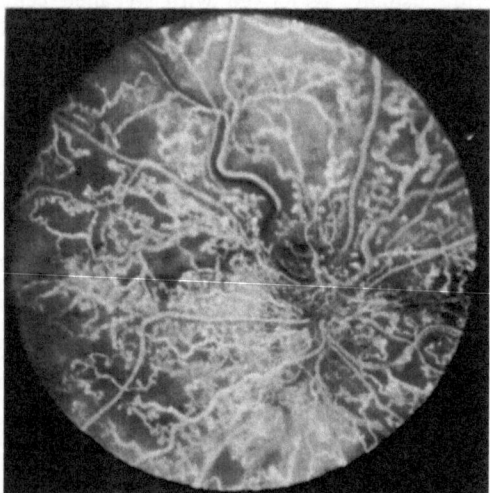

Fig. 2. Fluorescein fundus angiogram during retinal arteriovenous phase in a patient with hemorrhagic retinopathy.

in addition to venous statis; these angiographic appearances are not unique of hemorrhagic retinopathy bacause exactly identical changes are also seen

118

in many other conditions which include pulseless disease, (SHIMIZU,)
post-radiation retinopathy (HAYREH, 1970) diabetic retinopathy, Eales'
disease, sickle cell retinopathy, (GOLDBERG, 1971) incontinentia pigmenti
(WATZKE & STEVENS) retrolental fibroplasia — in the last four conditions
the changes usually start at the periphery of the retina. The common factor
in all these conditions and hemorrhagic retinopathy is ocular ischemia. Although the etiology of ischemia in all of them is different; in spite of that
the retinal vascular responses to ischemia is identical. Thus the angiographic
appeances of fully developed venous stasis retinopathy and hemorrhagic
retinopathy are completely different, the former showing evidence of venous stasis alone, and the latter that of retinal ischemia. The symptomatology, ophthalmoscopic appearances, prognosis and other features of the
two are also dissimilar and are summarized in Table I.
(WESSING & MEYER-SCHICKERATH; HAYREH)

The sequence of events in the pathogenesis of hemorrhagic retinopathy
most probably is as follows: Retinal arterial occlusion (partial or complete,
transistory or prolonged) leads to stasis of the retinal circulation, which in turn
produces venous stasis. The latter in already unhealthy and stenosed
central retinal veins (due to arteriosclerosis of the adjacent central retinal
artery, endothelial proliferation or presence of a partial thrombosis) precipitates thrombosis and completes occlusion of the central retinal vein;
thus this venous stasis acts as a triggering factor to complete the occlusion in
the vein.

After this, three processes take place:
1. Since some retinal arterial circulation is almost always restored within a
few hours or days, (HAYREH, 1971) it starts to fill the retinal vascular bed
with blood and also some blood enters the retinal vascular bed via the
anastomoses between the retinal and the optic disc vascular beds (the latter
is derived from the posterior ciliary artery circulation — Fig. 3).
2. Because of the complete block in the central retinal vein, the blood
cannot leave the retinal vascular bed.
3. The retinal ischemia also produces ischemic capillaropathy in the retinal
vascular bed. This capillaropathy renders the capillaries incapable of with-
standing a normal or high intracapillary pressure.

Under the combined influence of these three factors, the rise of intra-
luminal pressure in retinal capilaries produced by the perfusing blood causes
the retinal capillaries to rupture, resulting in hemorrhagic retinopathy. This
indicates that unless some retinal arterial circulation is restored, the fundus
is not likely to show any gross hemorrhages. Hence fluorescein angiography
would always show some arterial circulation in hemorrhagic retinopathy.

The role of intraocular pressure in the production of hemorrhagic retinopathy is important. This is because any factor which lowers the perfusion
pressure in the central retinal artery to a level lower than the intraocular
pressure would stop the arterial inflow into the retina. In arteriosclerotic
individuals with narrowed central retinal artery or its parent trunks (i.e.,
ophthalmic or carotid arteries), the perfusion pressure under ordinary circumstances may be just enough to maintain normal retinal circulation but a
fall of perfusion pressure in the central retinal artery due to systemic arterial
hypotension below the intraocular pressure would stop the arterial circula-

119

TABLE I

Comparison of Clinical Features of
Venous Stasis Retinopathy and Hemorrhagic Retinopathy

	Venous Stasis Retinopathy	Hemorrhagic Retinopathy
Age	Young adults and past middle age	More common in those past middle age
Symptoms	May have none or vague blurred vision	Always marked deterioration of vision
Visual acuity	May be normal or only mildly to moderately defective, rarely markedly defective	Markedly defective
Visual fields	Peripheral – normal; Central – normal or with a relative/absolute central scotoma	Peripheral – usually markedly abnormal; Central – almost always abnormal with a central scotoma
Ophthalmoscopy A. Early cases Retinal veins	Markedly engorged, turgid and tortuous	Markedly engorged, turgid and tortuous
Retinal hemorrhages	Vary from a few flame-shaped and punctate hemorrhages to a large number in central part and punctate in peripheral regions.	Central part covered with gross hemorrhages. Progressive during initial stages; less in periphery.
Cotton-wool spots	Rare	Very common
Optic disc	Hyperemic and may be edematous	Usually covered with hemorrhages and swollen
Macula	Normal or may show edema	Gross hemorrhages and edema
Retinal arterioles	Normal or arterio-sclerotic	Usually arteriosclerotic and narrow
B. Late cases (after about 6-9 months or longer) Retinal veins	Mildly to moderately engorged. Sometimes sheathed	Mildly to moderately engorged and frequently sheathed
Retinal hemorrhages	May be none or usually a few, mainly in the periphery	May be none or only a few

	Venous Stasis Retinopathy	Hemorrhagic Retinopathy
Retina	Normal	Frequently microaneurysms, dilated capillaries and neo-vascularization. May have pre-retinal or vitreous hemorrhages.
Optic disc	Normal or slightly hyperemic, with retino-ciliary veins	May be pale disc, usually with retinociliary veins
Macula	Normal or may show cystoid degeneration	Macular degeneration and pigmentary disturbances. Sometimes pre-retinal fibrosis

Fluorescein Fundus Angiography

	Venous Stasis Retinopathy	Hemorrhagic Retinopathy
1. Early cases	Retinal venous stasis, engorged capillaries, some microaneurysms. Fluorescein staining of retina, maximum along main veins. In macular edema, fluorescent macular star seen.	Retinal venous stasis, engorged capillaries and microaneurysms, masked by gross hemorrhages. May have delayed retinal arterial filling. Late fluorescein staining of the retina and main veins.
2. Late cases	Mild to moderate retinal venous stasis, retino-ciliary veins on optic disc and may have some microaneurysms. No neovascularization or obliteration of retinal capillaries.	Mild to moderate retinal venous stasis, retinociliary veins on optic disc, areas of retinal capillary obliteration, arteriovenous shunts, neovascularization, and microaneurysms. Late staining of retina and veins.
Prognosis	Good	Poor
Course	Self-limited	Progressive
Complications	Macular edema → cystoid macular degeneration → central scotoma	Macular degeneration, pre-retinal of vitreous hemorrhages, retinitis proliferans, thrombotic glaucoma
Pathologically	Central retinal vein occlusion with stasis	Red infarct due to central retinal vein occlusion with arterial ischemia
Treatment	If macular edema develops, systemic corticosteroids effective	Usually no treatment seems effective

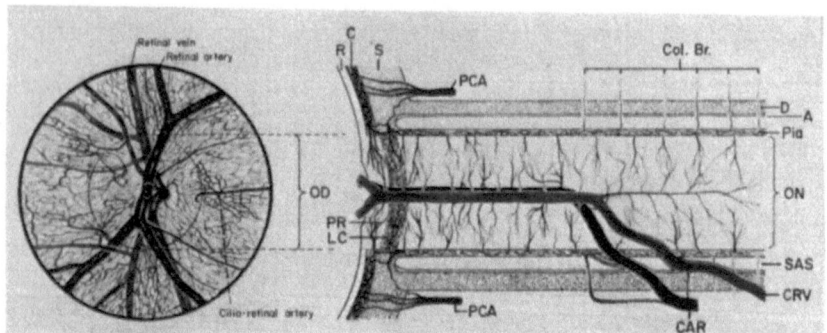

Fig. 3. Diagrammatic representation of the blood supply of the optic nerve.
Abbreviations

A	=	Arachnoid matter	OD	=	Optic disc
C	=	Choroid	ON	=	Optic nerve
CAR	=	Central retinal artery	PCA	=	Posterior ciliary artery
Col.Br.	=	Collateral Branches	PR	=	Pre-laminar region
CRV	=	Central retinal vein	R	=	Retina
D	=	Duramater	S	=	Sclera
LC	=	Lamina cribosa	SAS	=	Sub-arachnoid space

tion. Such a hypotension occurs during sleep. In hemorrhagic retinopathy the vast majority of patients notice marked deterioration of vision on waking one morning. In these frequently the retinal arterial circulation is restored with the restoration of normal systemic blood pressure in the course of the morning (as shown by fluorescein angiography), but retinal ischemia for a few hours during the night is enough to produce the above-mentioned retinal vascular changes, and produce hemorrhagic retinopathy on the restoration of the arterial circulation. The presence of a higher-than-normal intraocular pressure in arteriosclerotic individuals would make their eyes more prone to develop hemorrhagic retinopathy than those with normal intraocular pressure, because of the higher chances of developing imbalance between the perfusion pressure in the central retinal artery and intraocular pressure in these cases. In addition, raised intraocular pressure produces venous stasis by pressing the retinal veins on the optic disc.

In venous stasis retinopathy with the block in the central retinal vein situated behind the lamina cribrosa, anastomotic channels lying in the pre-laminar region of the optic disc connecting the central retinal vein with the chloroidal veins, are still patent and act as a safety valve mechanism to short circuit the blood from the central retinal vein to the chloroidal veins; the anastomotic channels enlarge with the passage of time to produce the re-tinociliary veins on the disc. If the thrombotic process involves the central retinal vein in the optic nerve head and also involves these anastomotic channels in the prelaminar region (Fig. 3), this would convert the retinal circulation into a closed circulation with no safety valve mechanism available. Under these circumstances, occlusion of the central retinal vein will produce secondary retinal arterial insufficiency because of the absence of any outlet for the blood. This was also demonstrated experimentally by FUJINO et al., (1969). This once again produces retinal arteriovenous occlusion and hemorrhagic retinopathy.

122

REFERENCES

FUJINO, T., CURTIN, V.T. & NORTON, E.W.D. Experimental central retinal vein occlusion. *Arch. Ophthal. (Chicago)*, 81: *395* (1969).

GOLDBERG, M.F. Classification and pathogenesis of proliferative sickle retinopathy. *Amer. J. Ophthal.*, 71: *649* (1971).

HAYREH, S.S. Occlusion of the central retinal vessels. *Brit. J. Ophthal.*, 49: *626* (1965).

HAYREH, S.S. Post-radiation retinopathy — A fluorescence fundus angiographic study. *Brit. J. Ophthal.*, 54: *705* (1970).

HAYREH, S.S. Pathogenesis of occlusion of the central retinal vessels. *Amer. J. Ophthal.*, 72: *998* (1971).

HAYREH, S.S. Central retinal vascular occlusion — Morphology and Pathogenesis. Proc. IX Internation. Congress Angiology, Florence, April 1974, Minerva Cardioangiologica, (In press).

HAYREH, S.S. Eales' disease. Proc. Int. Symp. Fluorescein Angiography, Albi, p. 680, Karger, Basel.

KEARNS, T.P. & HOLLENHORST, R.W. Venous stasis retinopathy of occlusive disease of the carotid artery. *Proc. Mayo Clinic*, 38: *304* (1963).

MICHEL, J. Die spontane Thrombose der Vena centralis des Opticus. *Albrecht v. Graefe's Arch. Ophthal.*, 24: *37* (1878).

SHIMIZU, K. Arterial and venous occlusions of the retina. Proc. IX Internation. Congres Angiology, Florence, April, 1974. Minerva Cardioangiologica (In press).

WATZKE, R.C. & STEVENS, T.S. Retinal vascular hypoplasia and telangiectasia associated with Incontinentia Pigmenti (Personal communication).

WESSING, A. & MEYER-S G. Fluorescein studies in Eales' disease and related lesions of the retina. Proc. Int. Symp. Fluorescein Angiography, Albi, pp. 608-612, Krager, Basel.

THE PATHOGENESIS OF RETINAL BRANCH VEIN OCCLUSION

I.C. MICHAELSON

(Jerusalem, Israel)

This condition results in a diffuse disturbance of the retinal capillaries, regional or general, with leakage of plasmoid transudate and hemorrhage into the retinal tissues. The clinical and histological findings and their frequent concurrence in one eye or in both eyes of the same patient indicate that the central and branch manifestations are varieties of the same condition. Because the branch variety appears ten times more frequently than central occlusion and is more capable of progressive observation, this report will be confined to it.

Apart from isolated cases based on abnormal blood states, two main general conceptions of the pathogenesis are:

1. The disease is directly due to vein stenosis, partial or complete, caused by the pressure of the overlying sclerosed artery at an arterial-venous crossing (Gunn's Sign), with resulting back-pressure effect on the capillary bed.

2. The disease, more complex in origin, is essentially due to a chronic arteriolar insufficiency associated with age, hypertension, or usually both; to a gradually resulting microcirculopathy which is finally hemorrhagic; and to one or more associated factors which further embarrass the microcirculation. These factors usually include a disturbed venous flow, the effect of stenosis of the vein at an a/v crossing; but may in addition frequently include the lowering of the general blood pressure as in sleep, a rise in intraocular pressure in glaucoma, or diabetes whose retinal pathology includes arteriolar narrowing and a severe microcirculopathy.

The main approaches to the elucidation of the pathogenesis of retinal vein occlusion have been as follows:

a. Ophthalmoscopy including fluorescein angiography.

b. Histological study of the a/v crossings in age and hypertension.

c. Study of enucleated or post-mortem eyes affected by vein occlusion.

There have been available many such eyes with central retinal vein occlusion because such eyes may be removed because of severe pain due to secondary glaucoma; but up till now, only three eyes with branch vein occlusion have been available for complete histological investigation.

d. Experimental production of the disease in animals (BECKER & POST, 1951; CAMPBELL, 1961; LINNER, 1961; HAYREH, 1965; FUJINO, 1969; KOHNER, 1970).

IMPEDIMENT AT ARTERIO-VENOUS CROSSING (GUNN'S SIGN)

The frequency with which Gunn's Sign is found in branch vein occlusion and the general impression of vein-nipping that this condition gives has resulted in a popular conception that venous occlusion is basically caused by venous flow impediment at the a/v crossing. SEITZ (1962) and BALLANTYNE & MICHAELSON (1970) have shown that this is by no means necessarily so; the former by demonstrating that the sign can be due to proliferation of the adventia of the vein at the crossing thus concealing the lumen but not constricting it, and the latter by showing that vein concealment may be due to retinal edema. There is, however, little doubt that at some Gunn's Signs there is a degree of impediment to the venous flow. In such cases, there is probably a banking of the vein distal to the crossing. It is not possible to determine clinically, even with the help of fluorescein angiography, whether an a/v crossing vein flow embarrassment is the basic cause or only an associated provoking cause. Histological examination of the a/v crossings in branch vein occlusion is rare and cannot necessarily help the elucidation. The determination of the role of vein stenosis is of obvious importance with regard to the feasibility of preventive therapy for retinal vein occlusion. Stenotic arterio-venous crossing changes are not likely to be helped by therapy.

CHRONIC INSUFFICIENCY OF ARTERIOLAR FLOW

Retinal vascular hypertension is characterized in its early phase by a narrowing of the arteriolar bed. In the course of time, however, there takes place a secondary fibrosis in the larger vessels near the disc which dilate in consequence of the increased intravascular pressures (LEISHMAN, 1957). This dilatation does not remain confined to the major arterioles but progressively affects the larger of the minor arterioles. In the course of a retinal vascular assessment of civil servants between 40-72 years of age, it was found that the average total minor arteriolar diameter in a group of hypertensives between 42 and 57 years of age was 524μ (MICHAELSON et al., 1966). However, as the result of the secondary arteriolar fibrosis and dilatation described, the average total minor arteriolar diameter in patients ranging from 58 to 72 years of age was 595μ. The arteriolar dilation is associated with increasing tortuosity of the vessel and enlargement of the angle of vessel division, which frequently becomes $90° - 180°$. In addition, the vessel light reflex becomes brighter and less soft. These arteriolar changes, noted histologically and clinically, most probably indicate a slowing arteriolar blood flow. RUBENSTEIN (1964) in fluorescein studies noted that the blood flow in the veins was unimpeded and concluded that arteriolar flow was deficient.

Arteriolar flow may be further embarrassed by the development of atheroma that begins in the larger vessels close to the disc. PATON (1964) found that 81 percent of 188 patients showed atheroma or hypertension. The intimal changes are patchy in distribution which is expressed clinically as calibre variation. Fatty degeneration in the proliferated intima may lead to sheating of the vessel. There is much clinical evidence of the role of atheroma in the pathogenesis of branch vein occlusion. The gross effect of atheroma on the vessel lumen in the histological reconstruction of a sheated vessel observed clinically and examined histologically (Fig. 1).

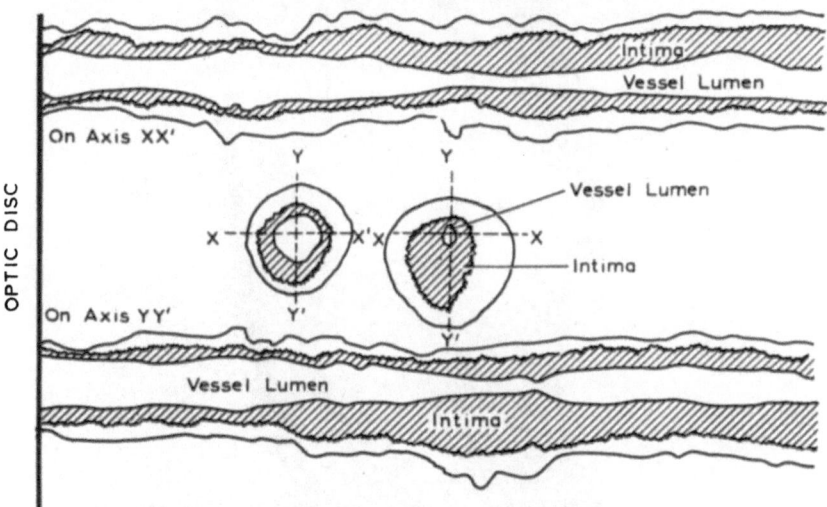

Fig. 1. Reconstructed longitudinal section of atheromalous vessel.

Occlusive carotid disease has been observed in 38 out of 1,300 unselected autopsies (HULTQUIST, 1942) and may give rise to a condition referred to as venous stasis retinopathy (KEARNS & HOLLENHURST, 1963). Retinal arteriolar pressure in this condition is found reduced on ophthalmodynamometry (COGAN, 1961; SMITH, 1964). The arterioles are narrowed, the veins engorged and there are numerous red dots of hemorrhages or micro-aneurysms alongside the vein. This condition may be amenable to treatment by endarterectomy (HERSKO & COLL, 1967).

Postmortem examination of the fundus was carried out in three eyes affected in four quadrants by branch venous occlusion or its imminence (RABINOWICZ et al., 1968). In all affected quadrants, the arterioles were grossly atheromatous while the veins were generally normal with respect to lumen diameter and wall thickness except at one a/v crossing (Fig. 2).

Reported experimental production of conditions similar to retinal vein occlusion has not taken into account the age or the general vascular state of the animal, parameters most important in the disease in humans. Most of the experiments have produced retinal hemorrhages following obstructive influences on the venous circulation produced by photocoagulation of the vessel trunk and the retinal tissues. These experiments do not appear to reflect what takes place in clinical and pathological experience. HAYREH (1965) succeeded in producing retinal hemorrhages following ligature of the central retinal vein only after ligaturing the central retinal artery as well.

It would appear that both arteriolar flow insufficiency and a degree of obstruction at an a/v crossing play a role in perhaps the majority of cases of branch vein occlusion (diagram). The problem as in other examples of mul-

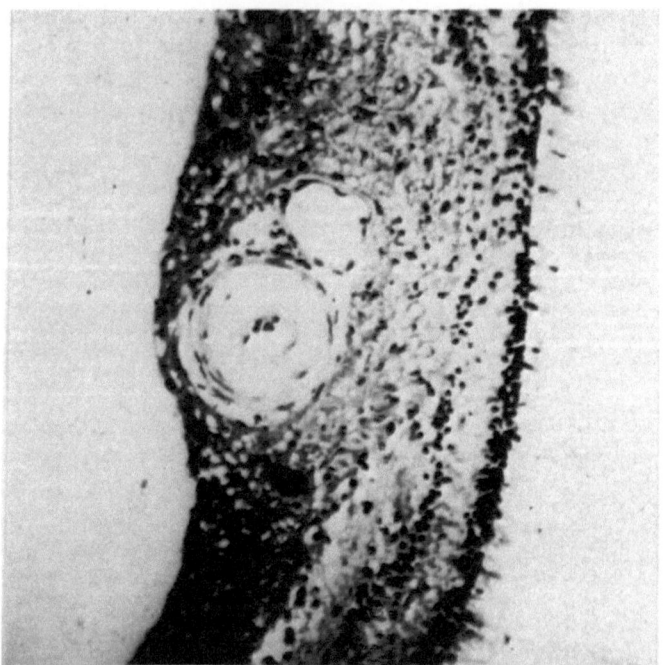

Fig. 2. Post mortem specimen showing very narrowed arteriole and wide-lumened vein within area of retina affected by branch vein occlusion

tiple causation in pathogenesis is to assess the causes, according to their relative frequency and degree. It frequently happens in branch retinal vein occlusion that there is an absence or very slight degree of obstruction at the a/v crossing as indicated by ophthalmoscopic and fluorescein appearances. On the other hand, there is nearly always a degree of disturbed arteriolar or arterial flow as described above. It would appear then that the diminished arteriolar flow is the primary and the more important element in the pathogenesis of retinal vein occlusion, with climactic associated factors, in cluding the vessel crossing flow impediment, temporary lowering of general blood pressure, increase of intraocular pressure or occasionally some increase in blood viscosity. Combined, these changes lead to a chronic retinal capillaropathy which may be local or general, and which may be nonhemorrhagic or hemorrhagic.

The following are the main disturbances of the capillary bed as evidenced on ophthalmoscopic, fluorescein or histological examination:

1. Stasis; indicated by capillary dilatation, venular dilatation, increase of capillary transit time.

2. Focal areas of capillary closure or defective filling; indicated, besides other evidence, by tortuous collateral circulation.

3. Retinal edema; perhaps indicated by Gunn's Sign besides other more obvious evidence. Edema may be present at the macula without hemorrhages (GASS, 1968).

4. Capillary degeneration; indicated by microaneurysms and hemorrhages, respectively circular or linear according to their origin from the deep or

128

superficial capillary layer.

The stages of branch venous occlusion may, therefore, be described as follows:

1. Arterial and arteriolar flow insufficiency.
2. Provoking associated factors.
3. Chronic microcirculopathy in a pre-hemorrhagic phase.
4. Chronic microcirculopathy in a hemorrhagic phase. (See Diagram).

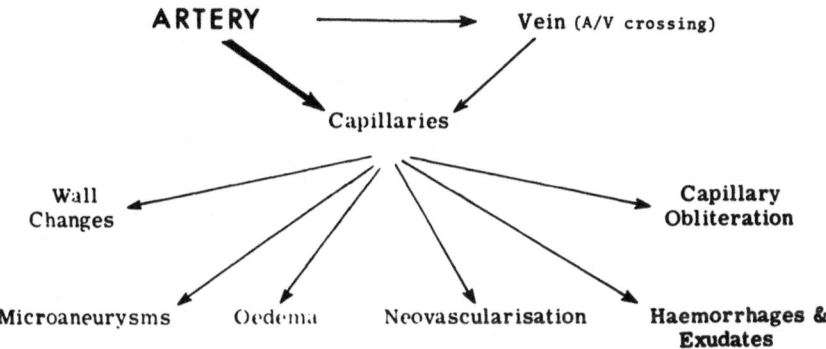

Diagram illustrating the pathogenesis of the capillaropathy in retinal branch vein occlusion. The relative rates of arteriolae flow insufficiency and a/v crossing impediment are indicated.

It is important that the pathogenetic stages of retinal vein occlusion be understood, because it is on the basis of this understanding that preventive measures can be devised; and it is on the basis of a common pathogenesis in retinal and cerebral occlusion that preventive measures found successful in one organ may be used with hopes of success in the other.

REFERENCES

BALLANTYNE, A.J. & MICHAELSON, I.C. Textbook of the Fundus of the Eye, 3rd edition, Edinburgh Livingstone, 1970.
BECKER, B. & POST, L.T. *Amer. J. Ophthal.*, 34: *677* (1951).
CAMPBELL, F.P. *Ophthal. (Chicago) Arch.*, 65: *2* (1961).
COGAN, D. *Arch. Ophthal.*, 66: *180* (1961).
FUJINO, T., CURTIN, V.T. & NORTON, E.W.D. *Arch. Ophthal.*, 81: *395* (1969).
GASS, J.D. *Arch. Ophthal.*, 80: *850* (1968).
HAYREH, S. *Brit. J. Ophthal.*, 49: *626* (1965).
HERSKO, C. & COLL, R. *Harefuah* 72: *344* (1967).
HULTOQUIET, G.T. Über Thrombose und Embolie der Arteria Carotid und hierbei vorkommende Gehirnveranderungen, Fischer, Jena, Stockholm, 1942.
KEARNS, T.P. & HOLLENURST, R.W. *Proc. Mayo Clinic* 38: *304* (1963).
KOHNER, E.M. *Amer. J. Ophthal.*, 69: *778* (1970).
LEISHMANN, R. *Brit. J. Ophthal.*, (1957).
LINNER, E. *Acta Ophthal.*, 39: *739* (1961).
MICHAELSON, I.C., ELIAKIM, AVSHALOM, A., MEDALIE, J.H., IVRY, M., & NEUMANN, E. 20th Intern. Ophthal. Cong., (1966).
PATON, RUBENSTEIN, I., & SMITH, U.H. *Trans. Ophthal. Soc. U.K.* 84: *559* (1964).
RABINOWICZ, I., LITMAN, S., & MICHAELSON, I.C. *Trans. Ophthal. Soc. U.K.* 88: *191* (1968).

RUBINSTEIN, K. *Trans. Ophthal. Soc. U.K.* 84: *564* (1964)
SEITZ R. *Klin. Mbl. Augenheilk.* 139: *491* (1962).
SMITH, V.H. *Trans Ophthal. Soc. U.K.* 84: *559* (1964)

REVIEW OF MEDICAL CONDITIONS ASSOCIATED WITH CENTRAL RETINAL VEIN OCCLUSION*

EVA M. KOHNER & J. CAPPIN

(London)

INTRODUCTION

Central retinal vein occlusion (CRVO) remains one of the most baffling problems in retinal vascular disease. Although the clinical features are well recognised, the pathogenesis remains uncertain. Nor is it obvious why some patients improve while others with apparently no more severe disease at the onset lose vision.

Over the years various medical conditions, in particular arterial diseases, have been thought to be responsible for the development of CRVO. In order to substantiate or refute the role of medical disorders we have examined 116 consecutive patients attending two London Hospitals with CRVO.

PATIENTS AND METHODS

During the years 1971-1973 all patients with CRVO attending the casualty department of Moorfields Eye Hospital (104 patients) and Kings College Hospital (12 patients) were referred for examination and were therefore unselected. The age and sex distribution of the patients is shown in Table I.

TABLE I.

AGE: (yrs)	Under 40	40 - 49	50 - 59	60 - 69	70 and Over	TOTAL
MALES	5	5	15	28	13	66
FEMALES	6	7	5	19	13	50
TOTAL	11	12	20	47	26	116

*This work was supported by the Wellcome Trust.

131

The majority of the patients were in the older age groups, but almost 10%, 11 patients, were under the age of 40 years.

Seventy-six of the patients were examined by one of the authors (EMK) while the other 40 were seen by the physicians of Moorfields Eye Hospital and Kings College Hospital.

Examinations and investigations were aimed towards finding possible factors of aetiological significance, haemoglobin, packed cell volume and serum proteins (to determine hyperviscosity states; viscosity itself was not measured) malignancy and arterial disease. Finally renal function was tested by estimating urine protein at clinic visits using Albustix and estimating blood urea. Serum creatinine was only measured in those with blood urea over 75 mg.%. Where possible the results were compared with population studies available.

RESULTS

a) Conditions associated with high blood viscosity

It is well known that high values of packed cell volume (PCV) are associated with high viscosity. Haemoglobin (Hb) concentrations reflect the PCV and the results obtained in the patients were compared with results of a population study carried out by CAMPBELL, GREEN, KEYSER, WATERS, WEDDELL & WITHEY (1968) in Wales. Figure 1 shows that

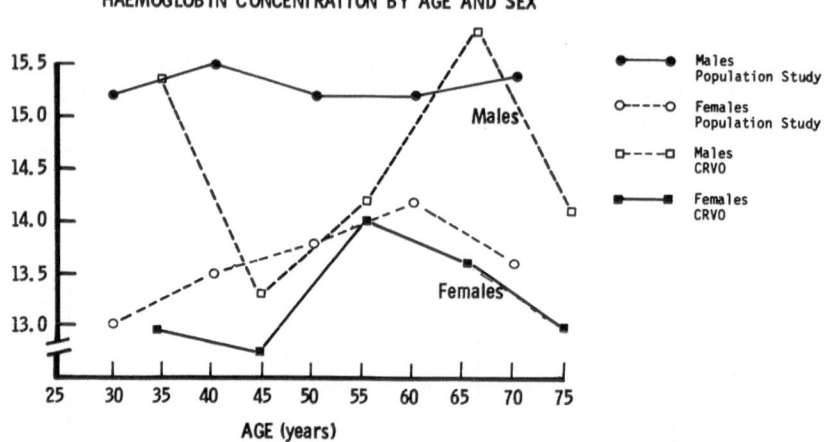

Fig. 1. Haemoglobin concentration by age and sex in patients with CRVO. (□ – □ males; ■ – females). The results of the population study of CAMPBELL et al. (1968) are plotted for comparison (● – ● males; ○ – ○ females).

similar to the general population male patients with CRVO had higher Hb levels than female patients but contrary to expectation the levels for both sexes tended to be lower than in the general population. This difference was most marked in the age group 40-49, where three of the male patients suffered from peptic ulcer. Two with severe anaemia (Hb under 9 g) were

132

not previously known to suffer from this condition.

In a sub-group of 35 patients detailed studies of blood clotting showed no abnormality.

None of the patients suffered from myeloma, cryoglobulinaemia or any of the paraproteinaemias causing increased blood viscosity. Minor abnormalities of serum proteins were present in 12 patients and included changes in α and β globulins mainly. These results do not suggest that an increased blood viscosity can be responsible for CRVO or affect its final outcome.

b. Malignancy

Previous work by Peart's group (ELLIS, HAMER, HUNT, LEVER, PEART & WALKER, 1964) indicated that malignancy, especially that of the large bowel, was common in CRVO. In this group of patients only 4 had malignant disease, one of the large bowel, one of the kidney, one of the prostate and one of the breast. This is not an unusually high number, and thus malignancy does not seem to be of importance in CRVO.

c. Arterial disease

Various aspects of vascular disease were found commonly in patients with CRVO (BRAENDSTRUP, 1950; KOHNER, 1964; RAITTA, 1965). It seemed to be essential to determine whether they were seen more commonly than in the general population and whether they affect the end result of the disease.

Diabetes — a condition associated with vascular disease — was only seen in 3 of the patients while 3 others had abnormalities of the glucose tolerance curve. Taking into account the age distribution of the patients there are probably no more diabetics among those with CRVO than in the general population.

Raised blood pressure is common in patients with retinal vein occlusion. Is it more common than in the population at large? Figure 2 compares the mean systolic and diastolic blood pressures in the group reported in the well known study of MIALL (MIALL & OLDMAN, 1958) In the Rhondda Fach and the Vale of Glamorgan. The striking feature is the close agreement of these results with those of Miall indicating that patients with CRVO do not differ greatly from those who do not have this disease.

Fasting serum cholesterol and triglycerides were studied in the patients. The results were compared with the recent report by LEWIS and his coworkers (1974) who studied a North London population. The mean serum cholesterol levels were similar in patients with CRVO and the normal population while triglycerides tended to be higher in most age groups. Taking arbitrary cut off points for both cholesterol and triglycerides at levels which are considered to be raised, it can be seen in Tables 2 and 3 that there are more patients with CRVO in these high lipid groups than members of the population study. Since raised lipids are associated with vascular disease this finding may prove to be of importance, but further studies will be needed to determine their exact role.

Serum uric acid levels, as expected, were higher in males than in females

133

FITTED CURVES RELATING SYSTOLIC AND DIASTOLIC PRESSURE
WITH AGE IN THE POPULATION SAMPLES

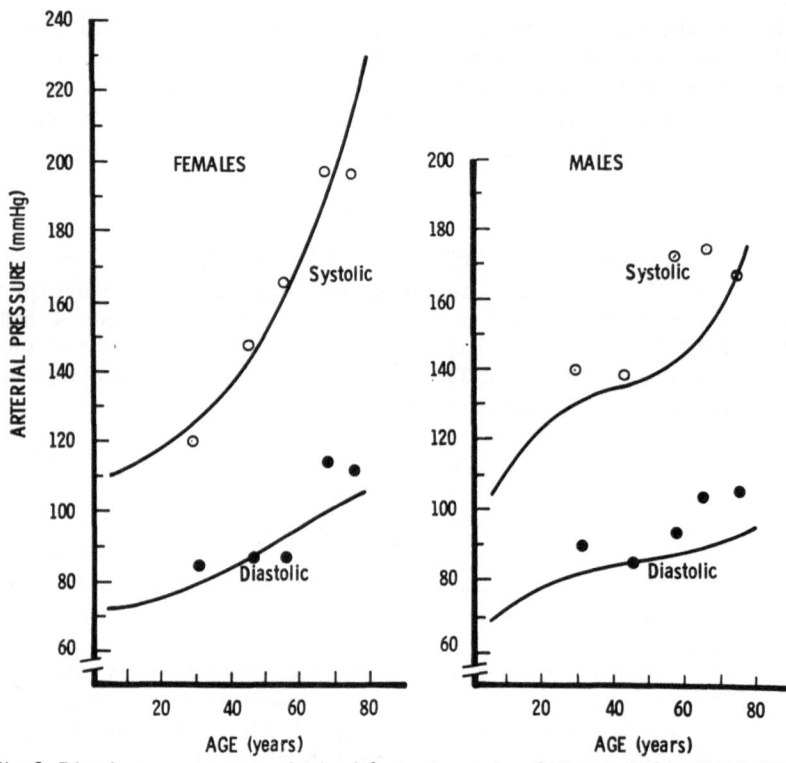

Fig. 2. Blood pressure curves obtained from the study of MIALL & OLDHAM (1958) with the results of the CRVO patients indicated by open circles for systolic and closed circles for diastolic pressures.

SERUM CHOLESTEROL

	Total No:	Over 320 mg/100 ml:		Over 280 mg/100 ml:	
POPULATION STUDY Men	142	2		15	
			$P < 0.005$		$P < 0.05$
C. R. V. O. Men	54	4		12	
POPULATION STUDY Women	146	0		15	
			$P < 0.005$		$P < 0.05$
C. R. V. O. Women	48	4		11	

SERUM TRIGLYCERIDES

	Total No:	Over 200 mg:	Over 180 mg:	Over 150 mg:
POPULATION STUDY Men	142	17	21	31
		P < 0.05	N.S.	P < 0.01
C. R. V. O. Men	54	9	14	23
POPULATION STUDY Women	146	2	4	7
		P < 0.05	P < 0.01	P < 0.005
C. R. V. O. Women	40	4	7	11

at all ages axcept those aged 70 and over. There were 23 patients, i.e. 1 in 5, whose uric acid was over 7 mg.%, the upper limit of 'normal' for our laboratory. This upper limit may be an under-estimation of that seen in the general population. In this group uric acid also failed to correlate with blood urea or Hb and fasting lipid levels.

d. Renal function

Finally renal function was tested by estimating urine protein at clinic visits using Albustix and estimating blood urea. Serum creatinine was only measured in those with blood urea over 75 mg.%.

Urine protein test was only positive in 5 patients, three of these had other evidence of renal impairment.

Blood urea in the group as a whole was not grossly different from the Welsh population studied by Campbell et al. (1968) except in the 60-69 age group where both males and females with CRVO appear to have higher blood ureas.

It is of interest that 3 patients had chronic renal failure with blood ureas 150-230 mg.% when first seen. This may indicate that renal disease of severe degree (or when chronic) is associated with an increased risk of thrombosis.

CONCLUSIONS

In this group of 116 patients no unique role for either arterial disease or any other medical condition could be found to account for occurrence of CRVO.

Chronic renal failure and raised serum lipids predisposing to arterial disease could have been responsible for the vascular occlusion in some of the patients. But apart from these two factors the important finding was how little this population differs from the general population.

It is of course possible that the presence of multiple predisposing factors are of greatest importance in the pathogenesis of CRVO — that will have to be studied in greater detail. However it is likely that in the majority of patients with vascular disease similar to that of the general population it is the local factors of intraocular pressure and other variables which determine the initial occurrence and visual outcome of CRVO.

135

REFERENCES

BRAENDSTRUP, P. *Acta Ophthal. Supp.*, 35: *1* (1950).
CAMPBELL, H., GREEN, W.J.W., KEYSER, J.W., WATERS, W.E., WEDELL, J.M. & WITHEY, J.L. *Brit J. prev. soc. Med.*, 22: *41* (1968).
ELLIS, C.J., HAMET, D.B., HUNT, R.W., LEVER, A.F., LEVER, R.S., PEART, W.S. & WALKER, S.M. *(Brit. med. Journal*, 2: *1093* (1964).
KOHNER, E.M. *Proc. roy. Soc. Med.*, 57: *816* (1964). LEWIS, B., CHAIT, A., WOOTTON, I.D.P., OAKLEY, C.M., KRIKKLER, D.M., SIGURDSSON, G., FEBRUARY, A., MAURER, B. & BIRKHEAD, J. *Lancet* 1: *141* (1974).
MIALL, W.E. & OLDHAM, P.D. *Clin. Sci.*, 17: *409* (1958).
RAITTA, C. *Acta Ophthal. Supp.*, 79-83: *12* (1965).

CEREBRAL STROKE, PATHOGENESIS
AND PREVENTIVE THERAPY

K.J. ZULCH

(Köln-Merheim, West Germany)

The pathogenesis of brain infarct is not yet fully analyzed and remains controversial.

The old clinical concept and term of thrombosis would indicate that in every case a local occlusion of a cerebral artery is responsible for a cerebrovascular attack (C.V.A.). However, it is well known that morphologically — both at autopsy as in the angiogram — between forty to sixty percent of the brain infarcts occur with open arteries. The same holds true for Transcient Ischemic Attacks. Experiences with coronary infarcts are similar (DOERR). This indicates that probably a hemodynamic factor plays a prominent role in the causation of the circulatory problem. The blood pressure seems to be the most important factor. However, other factors such as cardiac output, viscosity and oxygenation of the blood and the heart rhythm, are also of importance.

Since the majority of such cases shows an impairment of the supplying vessels by arteriosclerosis of the stenosing type, one could conceive that as a model a local 'stenosing factor' and a 'hypotensive crisis' of the blood pressure following cardiac failure or peripheral insufficiency are responsible for the local embarrassment of the circulation.

Actual occlusion remains a definite cause in the rest of the cases. Apart from stenosis of the arterial lumen by arteriosclerosis, other abnormalities like the 'ectatic' changes of the artery can lead to local impairment of the blood stream. Still other forms include kinking or coiling or external strangulation from the surrounding tissues as by osteochrondrotic osteophytes of the vertebrañ artery.

Statistics from vascular surgery indicate that a restriction of the lumen of an artery of 50 percent leads to a fall of peripheral arterial pressure and a restriction of 80 to 90 percent to an actual decrease of blood flow. These figures, however, are valid only where the blood pressure is normal. In hypotension, marked differences occur.

Morphological observations show that even with a complete occlusion of a supplying artery, a brain infarct may be missing. This suggests the possibility and efficiency or collateral circulation on the base of genuine anastomotic communications. However, if these anastomoses are not present at birth, they usually cannot be formed in the brain. This is in contrast to the pathophysiology of the heart.

However, in the 'four brain vessels' abundant anastomoses do occur in

137

the extra- and intracranial segments as shown by morphological observations and angiography.

Thrombosis may be primary. It may occlude the resting lumen of a highly stenosed artery and may also associated with thromboembolism.

Thrombosis may be dissolved within the first few days as proven by repeated angiography.

Finally, thrombosis may even be overcome without any permanent neurological changes. In these cases, the transient insufficiency of the existing collateral circulation can give rise to a 'Transient Ischemic Attack' (T.I.A.) or to a 'stroke'.

The basic pathologic principles that are at play may be summarized as follows:

1. Cerebral infarct follows occlusion of an artery if there is no collateral supply by preexisting anastomoses.

2. An infarct may be caused by a macroembolus, by primary or secondary thrombosis or by arteriosclerotic occlusion of an artery and by stenosis under unfavorable hemodynamic conditions, such as a hypertensive crisis.

3. There is a local predilection for arteriosclerotic stenosis and also for the thrombosis which are formed in these stenotic segments. The main cause of this being local 'turbulence'.

The foregoing are the classical concepts and are still accepted by the majority of scientists, yet a difference of opinion exists about the frequency of hemodynamic mechanisms. For the sake of completeness, two additional, different pathogenetic mechanisms causing ischemic cerebrovascular insufficiency must be considered:

The theory of microembolism: Ophthalmologists are familar with microemboli in the retina particularly those that follow amaurosis fugax. Vascular surgeons are of the opinion that microemboli are the causes of cerebrovascular accidents (C.V.A.'s), particularly in the form of Transient Ischemic Attacks (T.I.A.'s). Final proof of this theory awaits evidence from the pathologic laboratory.

The angiospastic insult: A second concept was derived from the classical interpretation of some C.V.A.'s precipitated by 'angiospasm' (angiospastic insult of V. BERGMANN & F. KAUFMANN). This concept was turned down by DENNY-BROWN (1951) in favor of the hemodynamic interpretation.

Recently, regional cerebral blood flow (RCBF) measurements of the Danish-Swedish groups have proved the value of the old Bayliss principle for the cerebral vessels: sudden induced hypertension ('hypertensive crisis') leads to a decrease of CBF. Since then, 'hypertension' has become one of the major concerns of the RCBF groups.

Practical examples will help illustrate these theoretical principles regarding the pathogenesis of cerebrovascular disturbances.

The efficiency of the ophthalmic artery as a collateral pathway will serve as an example. In case of an internal carotid occlusion, anastomoses via the three branches of the external carotid to the ophthalmic artery are in operation; they can fill retrogradely the syphon of the internal carotid artery, thus supplying great parts of the brain. Such anastomoses, if present and put into action by the necessary blood pressure can prevent infarction

138

in the area supplied by the internal carotid artery.

The modern hemodynamic concept of the 'last meadow' and of the 'frontier' or 'watershed' disturbances serve as additional examples.

Occlusion of one vertebral artery, which is half of the supply to the system of the basilar and posterior arteries, is not necessarily accompanied by severe neurological changes. Yet, frequently, severe neurological symptoms do occur. They originate from one of the six levels of the blood supply of the vertebrobasilar artery that nourish the medulla oblongata, pons, mesencephalon, thalamus, temporo-occipital lobe and the cerebellum. Symptoms of facial paresthesias, vertigo, vomiting, dysphagia, ataxia, or even as a single syndrome hemianopic defect may make their appearance.

Or else the disturbance can involve all six levels at the same time; however, then only parts of each area according to the principle of the 'last meadow'. This is a hemodynamic principle which explains why the most distant parts of a supply area are the first to be compromised in cases of vascular insufficiency.

The various patterns of a complex vascular system of circulation determine the position and size of the infarct after a given occlusion of one of the supply arteries. We have studied these patterns in the last ten years in the carotid system (ZULCH & GESSAGA, 1972) and in the vertebrobasilar area (METZINGER & ZULCH, 1971).

Moreover, there may be other patterns for the particular distribution of the area of insufficiency or infarct that is, for instance, the site of the occlusion in the various segments of the major intracranial arteries. In our department, DR. V. EINSIEDEL-LECHTAPE and Dr. HENNEMANN have studied the site of the occlusion of the posterior cerebral artery in relation to the subsequent infarct. At this artery one can define four types of occlusion:

1. A proximal block at the origin of the artery

2. A more distal block at the penduncular course, i.e., at the origin of the posterior communicating artery.

3. A further distant block at the summit of the peduncular circle of the posterior cerebral artery and

4. A distal occlusion at the branchings of the posterior cerebral artery.

Finally, as the fifth type one can have bilateral posterior occlusions at any of the points described above.

Morphologically, three gross types of infarcts may be distinguished in the posterior supply area: a. total infarct from the ammons horn down to the occipital pole, 2. proximal infarct dominantly in the temporo-occipital area and 3). 'infarct' in the 'center of the supply area'.

These various types of occlusions of the posterior cerebral artery are the result of an action of the so-called meningeal anastromoses of Heubner, coming from the anterior and middle cerebral arteries. They can play a prominent role in supplying part or the majority of the area endangered by the proximal occlusion. 'Central' infarcts of the posterior supply area may lead to clear-cut hemianopia or, if bilateral, even to amaurosis.

Infarcts in the territory of the posterior cerebral artery comprise around 10 percent of all cerebral infarcts, yet 80 percent of the patients with posterior infarcts have multiple cerebral infarction. The average age is around 70 years. However, two-thirds of the infarcts are old and already cystic, which reduces the value of this information.

In almost 50 percent of the cases, the total area striata is infarcted. In the majority, the infarct is more proximal and the distal part — the occipital pole is affected only in one-third of the cases.

Since a lower part of the area striata is more commonly compromised by the infarct than the upper, the more common clinical symptom of an upper quadrant hemianopia can be readily explained. The occipital pole, where the representation of central vision is very near, may get a particularly good supply by the Heubner's leptomeningeal anastomoses from the anterior and middle cerebral arteries as already stated more than 100 years ago by ROBERT FORSTER.

As a last example of hemodynamic studies (ZULCH, 1971) on problems of vascular insuffieicny, there is loss of vision or even amaurosis of one or both eyes after profuse loss of blood elsewhere in the body. This could be easily explained by the vascular architecture of the retina, if one adopts the hemodynamic principles of brain and spinal cord infarct. Central vision corresponds to an area which is 'the last field' for all the small nutrient arteries coming from outside radially to the macula. This may be compared to the spinal segment, where similar hemodynamic conditions prevail in central necrosis (ZULCH, 1954, 1967).

Venous compromises of the brain may not have the same importance as those in the retina (ZULCH, 1966). It is possible that it is more difficult to distinguish the exact primary vessel that is responsible. It is further possible that even in the retina, disturbances are more commonly hemodynamic and even primarily on the arterial side. The venous changes follow and later assume the predominant role.

There is one interesting phenomenon which has not been sufficiently investigated until recently. This is the difference in the course of the cerebral veins. Near the midline of the base in the old 'deep' parts of the neural tube, i.e., in the basal ganglia, the midbrain, pons and oblongata, veins run parallel to the arteries. In all the other 'superficial' parts of the brain, the veins have a different pattern from that of the arteries and drain into the sinuses. This difference in the course of the cerebral arteries in the hemispheric mantle and the great veins and sinuses is causing the considerable distance of the arteries from the veins on the surface. Therefore, the pattern of arterial and venous disturbances is easy to distinguish. Perhaps in the basal ganglia where arteries and veins are very close and run parallel, their proximity may comprise each other.

Occlusion of the superior sagittal sinus in contrast leads to venous disturbances or even infarcts in the draining area of the 'bridging veins'. This leads to heavy edematous transudation of great parts of the frontoparietooccipital brain adjacent to the sinus.

Occlusion of the right transverse sinus can produce a diffuse edema since this sinus drains in two-thirds of the cases the whole brain mantle. A subsequent unilateral or bilateral sixth nerve paresis, the so-called 'Gradenigo Syndrome' in the 'otitic hydrocephalus' of CHARLES SYMONDS, can occur.

1. Preventive therapy of stroke is preventive therapy of cerebral arteriosclerosis.

2. Preventive therapy of stroke is prevention and treatment of cardiac involvement and also that of arteriosclerosis of the coronary vessels.

3. A very prominent factor is blood pressure and as a vis-a-vis relationship. In rare cases it may act as a 'hypertensive crisis', in the majority of cases the 'hypotensive crisis' in labile hypertension or even in normo- or hypotension may be the cause of cerebrovascular disturbances.

4. Local stenosis in the carotid vertebral artery leading to T.I.A.'s may be surgically approached.

5. Therapy of beginning or progressive stroke is essential therapy for disturbances of vital functions. They require intensive type of care that includes cardiovascular therapy, maintenance of blood pressure, prevention of the edema, red blood cell aggregation or elevation of viscosity, vaso-active treatment, and general care of the patient.

REFERENCES

BERGMANN, G.V. Funktionelle Pathologie, Kap. 12: Die Lehre von der Apoplexie. Springer-Verlag, Berlin, 1932.

DENNY-BROWN, D. The treatment of recurrent cerebrovascular symptoms and the question of 'vascopasm.' *Med. Clin. N. Amer.*, 35: *1457-1474* (1951).

DOERR, W. Plotzlicher Herztod — Morphologische Aspekte. In: *Verh. Dtsch. Ges. Inn. Med.*, 78: *944-969* (1972).

FORSTER, R. Über Rindenblindheit. *Arch. Ophthal.*, 36: *94-108* (1890).

KAUFFMANN, Fr. Klinisch-experimentelle Untersuchungen zum Krankheitsbild der arteriellen Hypertension. *Z. exper. Med.*, 42: *473-495*; 43: *141-169* (1925) und *Z. Klin. Med.*, 1925: 100.

METZINGER, H. & ZULCH, K.J. Vertebro-basilar occlusion and its morphological sequelae. In: Cerebral Circulation and Stroke, edit. by K.J. ZULCH, pp. 67-81. Springer-Verlag, Berlin-Heidelberg-New York, 1971.

SYMONDS, CH. Hydrocephalic and focal cerebral symptoms in relation to thrombophlebitis of the dural sinuses and cerebral veins. *Brain* 60: *531-550* (1937).

ZULCH, K.J. Mangeldurchblutung an der Grenzzone zweier Gefäßgebiete als Ursache bischer ungeklarter Rückenmarksschadigungen. *Dtsch. Zschr. Nervenhk.*, 172: *81-101* (1954).

ZULCH, K.J. Neurologische Diagnostik bei endokraniellen Komplikationen von otorhinologischen Erkrankungen. *Arch. Ohren-Nasen-Kehlophk.*, 183: *1-85* (1964).

ZULCH, K.J. La circulation cérébrale: étude physio-pathologique. Symposion International sur la Circulation Cérébrale, Paris, 1965. Sandoz Edit. Paris, 1966.

ZULCH, K.J. Die spinale Mangeldurchblutung und ihre Folgen. Diskussion. *Verh. Dtsch. Ges. Inn. Med.*, 72: *1007-1059* J.F. Bergmann, Verlag, Munchen, 1967.

ZULCH, K.J. Some basic patterns of the collateral circulation of the cerebral arteries. In: Cerebral Circulation and Stroke, edit. by K.J. ZULCH. Springer-Verlag, Berlin-Heidelberg-New Yorkm 1971, pp. 106-122.

ZULCH, K.J. & GESSAGA, E. Infarcts in the carotid system. *Vascular Surgery* 6: *114-119* (1972).

CLINICAL ASPECTS OF RETINAL VEIN OCCLUSION OF SIGNIFICANCE FOR THE UNDERSTANDING OF ITS PATHOGENESIS, THERAPY OR PREVENTION

S. MERIN & M. IVRY

(Jerusalem, Israel)

The exact pathogenesis of retinal vein occulsion, branch or central is still a controversial subject. Various factors can be blamed as causing retinal vein occlusion. Among them is insufficiency of arterial blood flow caused by a primary disease of the artery, or by changes in the blood components. Further, a slowing down of the blood flow could be associated with capillary pathology. Finally, impediment of the venous flow can be caused by pressure on the vein at the A/V crossing or at the lamina cribrosa.

We would like to suggest that the clinical examination of a patient with retinal vein thrombosis by ophthalmoscopy and fluorescein angiography frequently reveals one or more of these underlying causes. Eight patients will be briefly presented to illustrate this point.

Some patients show signs indicating an impediment to the venous flow. In a patient with branch vein occlusion, whose fundus is shown in Fig. 1

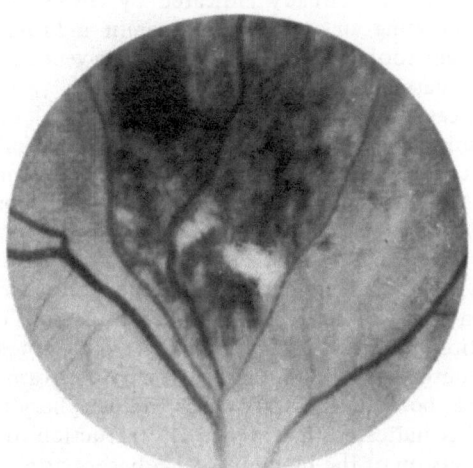

Fig. 1. Branch Vein Occlusion (see text).

the hemorrhages and exudates started at the point where the branch vein crosses the artery and were sharply bound by the two adjacent arterial

143

branches. This distribution of the hemorrhages in a sector served by one vein indicates an actual impediment to the flow in the vein at the apex of this triangular sector. Venous blood from inside this triangle is drained only by the affected vein. Outside the arteries, on both sides the drainage is through adjacent veins.

In another patient with lower temporal branch vein occlusion (Fig. 2)

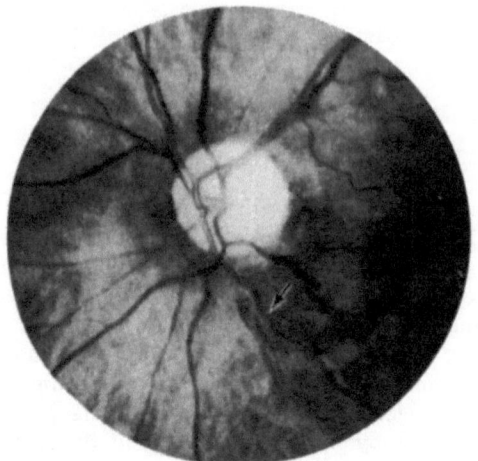

Fig. 2. Branch Vein Occlusion. The arrow indicates the presumably occluded A/V crossing.

veno-venous anastomoses around an arterio-venous crossing near the disc margin could be seen. As already indicated by GASS, such anastomoses around an A/V crossing or at the disc margin indicate that an actual occlusion of the vein took place at this point. The venous blood flow finds new channels to bypass the point of obstruction.

Similarly, in a case of central vein thrombosis (Fig. 3), one year after the event, venous retino-ciliary anastomoses on the disc indicate an actual impediment to the venous flow, probably at the lamina cribrosa. This caused the blood flow to be diverted around the point of obstruction. Please note that the arteries are abnormal as well, showing prominent caliber variations (arrow).

In a patient with a small branch vein occlusion, fluorescein angiography showed a delay in filling of the vein up to an arteriovenous crossing (Fig. 4). In the recirculation phase several veno-arterial anastomoses can be seen linking the obstructed vein to the adjacent arterioles (arrows). The artery from here onwards became thicker towards the periphery and its color was venous. Again, this indicates that an actual obstruction of the vein at this point caused a diversion of the blood into an adjacent artery.

Sometimes, the sign of an arterial involvement are the most pronounced.

In a patient with posterior superior temporal branch vein thrombosis (Fig. 5), ophthalmoscopy and fluorescein angiography revealed severe arteriolar pathology as the predominant finding. In such cases it is

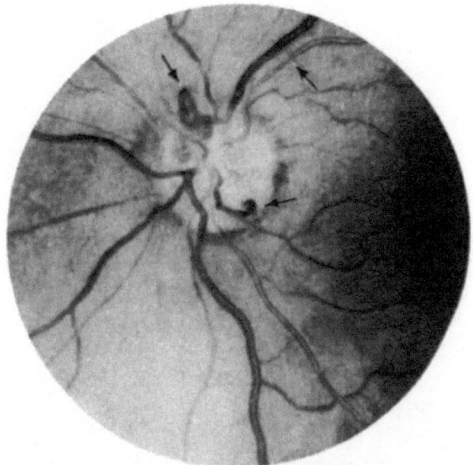

Fig. 3. Central retinal vein occlusion. The right upper arrow points to an arteriole with caliber variations. The other arrows point to retino-cilliary anastomoses.

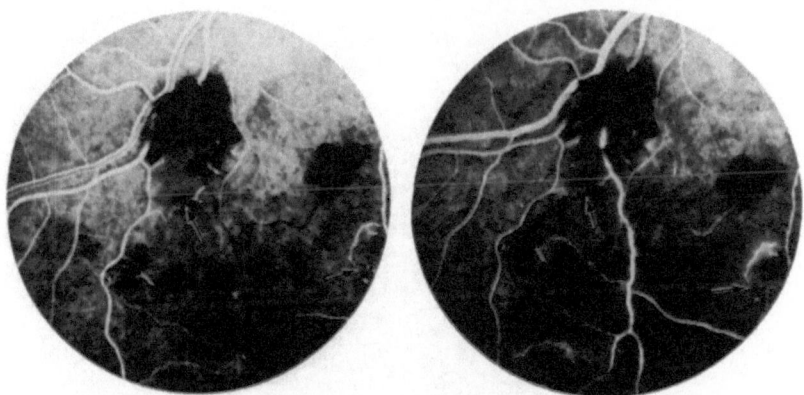

Fig. 4. Branch vein occlusion fluorescein angiography. A — arterio-venous phase; B — recirculation phase. Arrows indicate veno-arterial anastomoses.

impossible to decide what was the primary abnormality. However, the so often seen severe arteriolar involvement with practically normal veins in cases of venous occlusion, as in this case, might indicate a primary role of arteriolar pathology.

In another patient with posterior branch vein thrombosis (Fig. 6) ophthalmoscopy revealed severe arteriolar pathology in the involved area. Fluorescein angiography showed an arterio-arterial anastomosis, indicating that arteriolar obstruction might have been the primary cause of the disease.

Fluorescein angiography reveals in many cases signs of extensive capillary involvement.

The next patient had an inferior temporal vein thrombosis. Fluorescein angiography showed tortuous and abnormal capillaries all around the macula with leakage in the recirculation phase, including areas distant from

145

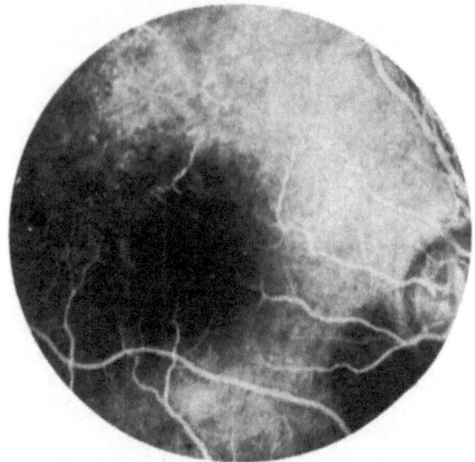

Fig. 5. Superior temporal branch vein occlusion. Severe pathology of branches of superior temporal artery above the macula.

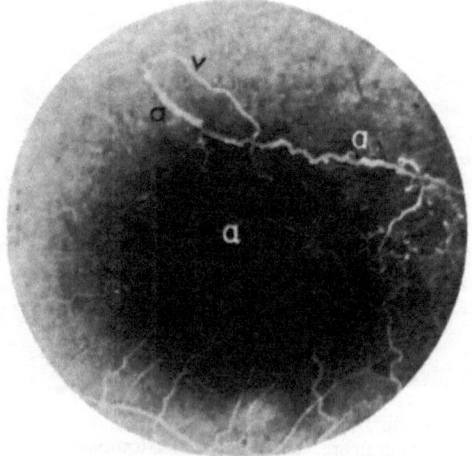

Fig. 6. Post branch vein occlusion. A – arterioles, V – venules.

the involved quadrant.

A 32-year-old juvenile diabetic, without diabetic retinopathy, suddenly developed a typical central retinal vein thrombosis (Fig. 7). The fluorescein angiogram, done shortly after the event showed capillary pathology and spots of leakage. This case illustrates the widespread capillary pathology seen in a systemic disease predisposed to vein thrombosis.

The fluorescein angiograms described above were performed a couple of days to a few months after the first clinical symptoms appeared. At this time, primary and secondary changes may both be seen in the affected eye and it may be difficult to distinguish one from another. Nevertheless, as shown here, a study of each case can suggest the early pathological changes which took place.

146

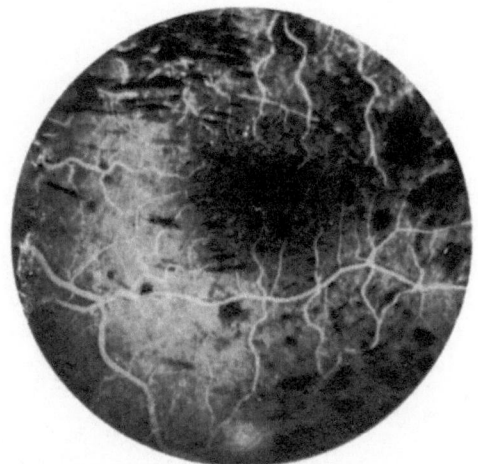

Fig. 7. Central retinal vein occlusion in a juvenile diabetic.

In most cases a combination of all the mentioned findings can be seen. This would, at least on clinical grounds, implicate both arterial and venous pathology as a combined cause of retinal vein occlusion. Insufficient blood inflow usually due to arterial, arteriolar or capillary disease and an actual obstruction on the venous side combine to cause the typical picture.

CLINICAL ASPECTS OF RETINAL VEIN OCCLUSION SIGNIFICANT FOR THE UNDERSTANDING OF ITS PATHOGENESIS AND PREVENTIVE THERAPY

K. RUBENSTEIN

(Birmingham, England)

In spite of being ophthalmoscopically spectacular, clinically frequent, pathologically studied for nearly a century and reported as a distinct syndrome since the work of VON MICHEL in 1878, retinal vein occlusion still presents problems all along the line. We are in doubt about the diagnosis itself as witnessed by the recurring attempts to isolate the real phlebitis from the syndrome. We are in doubt about histopathology because true thrombosis, endothelial proliferation and embolisation and inflammation of the veins were in the past demonstrated by some but denied by others who found no trace of occlusion of the veins in cases presenting the clinical fundus picture. We are in doubt etiology, the old assumptions about underlying focal infection and chronic granulomata being replaced by knowledge that a host of blood dyscrasias and vascular insufficiencies in the carotid system, including surgical ligations, may produce a fundus picture of vein occlusion. No wonder that we still neither know how to treat it nor do we know how to prevent it.

The problems of interpretation of a clinical picture of retinal vein occlusion – central or branch – are three: the mechanisms of peripheral fundus hemorrhages, the pathogenesis, and the etiology.

MECHANISM

Until the advent of fluorescein angiography of the retina, the only guides to the understanding of the fundus picture were histological studies. The material available for these studies consisted mainly of the eyes enucleated because of vitreous hemorrhage and a secondary glaucoma. Two opposing conclusions were outstanding: first that the process is that of true thrombosis of the vein and second that the basic pathological changes center on endothelial proliferation; Further microscopic studies revealed that in many cases neither of these could be found at all. More recently, meticulous histological studies of SEITZ (1961) failed to demonstrate mechanical compression of the veins either. Histological examination of three cases of clinically observed vein branch occlusion were reported by RABINOWICZ and others (1968): extensive arterial degeneration but patency of 'affected' veins – except one – were demonstrated. Fluorescein studies from the very start showed slowing of the dye passages but obvious patency of the

149

'occluded' veins in all early cases. (RUBENSTEIN, 1964). Coupled with observations of very similar fundus pictures in various diseases known to slow or diminish circulation in the retina, the conclusions seem to be unescapable that the picture of the vein occlusion is that of stasis.

PATHOGENESIS

The pathogenesis of this stasis in the majority of idiopathic cases of retinal vein occlusion has been considered in the past to rest on the mechanical slowing of venous outflow at the point of exit of the veins from the eye — lamina cribrosa — in central vein occlusion and/or at the arterio-venous crossings by a sclerosed arteriole in branch occlusion. Experimentally one can produce a picture of branch vein occlusion by the use of Argon Laser (HAMILTON et al., 1974). Histopathological studies of clinical cases failed to demonstrate such occlusions and fluorescein angiography clearly showed slowing of the passage of dye in the veins centripetally and not its banking at the side of assumed obstruction. Moreover, fluorescein studies demonstrated a marked degree of degeneration of the venous walls which stain with the dye and allows it to leak into the retinal tissue along various segments of the veins, not at the suspect arterio-venous crossings. In general diseases presenting vein occlusion fundus picture, the reasons for slowing of blood flow are well known. In carotid artery insufficiency, or aortic artery syndrome or artery ligation, the cause is the diminished bulk of blood reaching the retinal arterioles. In disproteinaemias the viscosity of blood is increased because of excess of Gamma globulins. In sickle cell anemia, the distorted red cells mechanically block the arteriolar branches. In polycythaemia these branches are blocked by excess of red cell corpuscles. In all these conditions the slowing of the blood is caused by bloackage at the arteriolar and not venous side of circulation watershed. The majority of idopathic retinal vein occlusions do not belong to any of these etiologically understood diseases. Here, however, the common denominator is clearly the arteriolar involution. Histologically, the presence of arteriolar sclerosis has been the one constant feature found in all specimens studied. Clinically the involvement of retinal arterioles was observed from the earliest days of recorded ophthalmoscopic observations. In rhesus monkey experiments it was shown that the closure of the central retinal vein behind the lamina cribrosa did not produce a fundus picture of vein occlusion, but if the accompanying artery is occluded as well, the picture developed (HAYREH, 1964). Clinically, the vein occlusion picture develops when there is a gradual impairment of blood flow through the arterioles. A sudden arrest will manifest itself as a classical arterial occlusion.

Contrary to the then held opinion, our own studies demonstrated visual field changes in 84 percent of a consecutive series of 120 cases (RUBINSTEIN, 1964) and 64 percent were — mostly sectorial — typical for arterial occlusions. We also demonstrated in 75 percent, sheathing, cuffing and the presence of plaques on the arteriolar walls of the involved sectors. Primary arteriolar involution may affect the blood flow through the veins in two ways: either by simple denial of normal volume of blood or by involvement of the companion veins in the adventitial hypertrophy of the arteriolar

150

walls at the arterio-venous crossings. This hypertrophy could lead to the narrowing of the venous lumen. It is quite probable that either of these mechanisms is in operation in different patients depending on the anatomical and pathological state of the vessels.

ETIOLOGY

Regarding the etiology of arterial changes in retinal vein occlusions, there are clearly two factors involved. First the average age of patients affected is 60 which points strongly to the role of senile involution. The second feature is the presence of hypertension in two-thirds of the patients (RUBINSTEIN & JONES, 1974). It seems that while the aging process is the main physiological feature, hypertension, not necessarily severe, is the main pathological feature. The usual good therapeutic results that occur in cases of marked hypertension where the blood pressure can be brought down by appropriate medication seem to support this view. This is to be contrasted with the usual failure to influence the state of the retinal circulation by anticoagulant and fibrinolytic agents, not mentioning even the failure of treatment by corticosteroids. There are no thrombi or signs of inflammations. With the usual etiological background of generalized arteriolar involution reversal back to normal of the affected circulation could not be seriously expected except on rare occasions. My own studies on the effect of low molecular Dextran to facilitate the retinal blood flow are not yet at the stage to allow conclusions.

PREVENTION

If we are right in apportioning the etiological role to hypertension and arteriolar involution then the prospects of prevention become uncertain. The changes concerned are those of wear and tear connected in many cases with the aging process. The level of hypertension that would justify treatment is not quite established. Diastolic blood pressure of around 100 may be sufficiently significant and should perhaps be treated before the retinal vascular changes destroy the vision.

CLINICAL ASPECTS OF RETINAL BRANCH VEIN OCCLUSION SIGNIFICANT FOR THE UNDERSTANDING OF ITS PATHOGENESIS AND PREVENTIVE THERAPY*

EVA M' KOHNER, J.S. SHILLING & R.S. CLEMETT

(London, England)

In 1964 PATON, RUBENSTEIN & SMITH presented a paper at the Ophthalmological Society for the United Kingdom in which they showed pictures of retinal branch vein occlusion (RBVO) associated with arterial disease in the same retinal quadrant. They concluded that the clinical picture of RBVO was due to arterial occlusion (i.e. retinal 'ischaemia') rather than vein occlusion. Indeed, they doubted the existence of vein occlusion, since in most instances perfusion of veins was evident. Their theory appeared to be supported by experimental work on central vein occlusion by HAYREH (1965).

In this short communication we hope to show that although arterial disease is probably of aetiological significance in the common 'classical' type of RBVO and often co-exists in the frequently seen 'diabetic' type; arterial occlusion is not responsible for the clinical picture well known to ophthalmologists.

CLASSICAL RETINAL BRANCH VEIN OCCLUSION

1. Aetiology

a). Arterial disease

In order to establish the role of arterial disease we have assessed its incidence in a series of patients with RBVO attending Moorfields Eye Hospital between 1972-1974.

The first 120 have now been analysed and the following findings recorded:

Raised blood pressure alone (above 160/100 mm.Hg.)	75
Hyperlipidaemia alone (serum cholesterol over 280 mg and/or fasting triglycerides over 150/100 ml)	13
Both raised blood pressure and hyperlipidaemia	18
Other vascular disease	3
Total	109

This table confirms that the presence of arterial disease is likely in a high proportion of patients. This finding is further emphasized by the site of the

*This work was supported by the Wellcome Trust.

occlusion, which is almost invariably at an arterio-venous crossing.

None of the patients had any evidence of arterial emboli at the time of presentation. More peripheral occlusion of some arterial branches was seen at the time of the first visit in a few patients, usually in those who presented more than 3 months after their first visual symptoms.

Many of the patients showed narrowing of veins at arterio-venous crossings (grade II hypertensive retinopathy of KEITH-WAGNER & BARKER, 1939) in other quadrants.

b). Venous disease

Complete occlusion of the vein at the arterio-venous crossing is seen only rarely while narrowing of the vein is common (Fig. 1a). That the venous

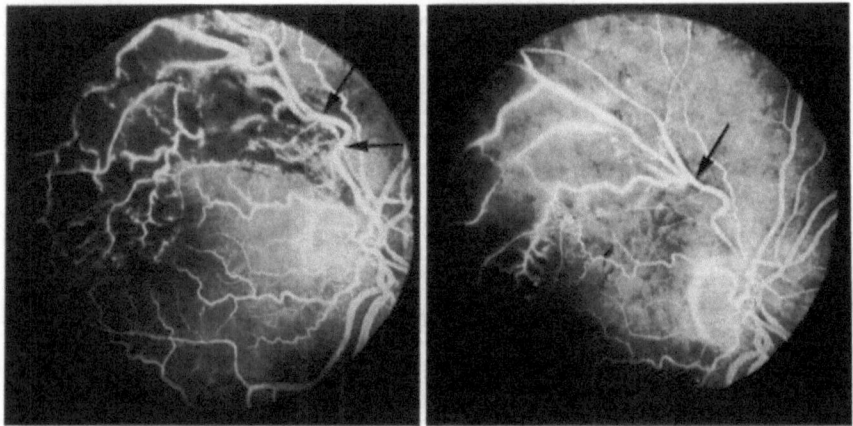

Fig. 1a. Fluorescein angiogram showing RBVO in superior temporal quadrant. Note arrowing of vein at the arterio-venous crossings (arrows).
b. Same as Fig. 1a. but 9 months later. Note disappearance of venous segment proximal to arterio-venous crossing (arrow).

wall is diseased and may have been occluded at least transiently or partially has been shown in post-mortem specimens by NEUBAUER (1960) and SEITZ (1963) and in life by SEITZ (1963) and CLEMETT (1974). CLEMETT (1974) demonstrated transient leakage of fluorescein from the veins at the site of the arterial crossing (Fig. 2a & b) in a high proportion of patients presenting within 6 weeks of their first symptom, in a few presenting within 6 weeks to 3 months, but in none who presented later. This finding emphasises the transient nature of venous wall disease. It is obvious that the occlusion is not permanent; it is probable that it does not have to be complete, since the retinal vasculature is already diseased and the ability to develop effective collaterals therefore impaired. Thus even partial or temporary occlusion can upset the precarious balance between in and outflow in these vessels.

That the clinical picture can occur in the absence of overt arterial disease is demonstrated by those few patients in whom no evidence of such disease

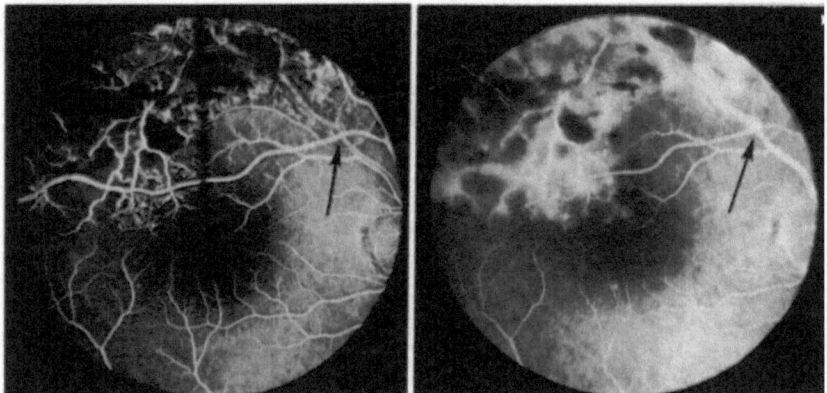

Fig. 2a. Fluorescein angiogram of RBVO 6 weeks after first visual symptom showing arterio-venous crossing, site of occlusion (arrow).
b. Same as Fig. 2a. but few seconds later. Nore leakage of fluorescein at the site of occlusion (arrow).

can be found.

Experimental work reported by KOHNER et al. (1970) and more recently by HAMILTON et al. (1974) also indicate that the full clinical picture of retinal branch vein occlusion including cotton wool spots can be produced by selective occlusion of retinal veins without damaging the arterial supply to the territory.

How, then, can the findings of PATON et al. (1964) be explained? A study of the natural history of RBVO in our series hopes to explain this dichotomy of opinion.

2. Results of Retinal Branch Vein Occlusion

a). Progressive venous changes

Immediately following RBVO there is dilatation and leakage of fluorescein from the vein distal to the occlusion. Later whole segments of the vein may disappear (Fig. 1a & b) and peripheral venous segments may get non-perfused. Another feature seen not uncommonly is reduplication of veins. This occurs usually at the site of occlusion or narrowing of the vein. It is unlikely to be the result of simple recanalisation, since the reduplicated veins diameters are greater than those of the original vessels. It is probable that reduplication is a form of by-pass or collateral formation.

b). Progressive arterial changes

In experimental RBVO HAMILTON et al. (1974) observed arterial changes *following* the vein occlusion, though at the time of the vein occlusion there was no evidence of arterial disease. In several patients we were able to follow the progressive narrowing and development of sheathing and irregularity of the arteries many months after the vein occlusion. In some patients peripheral parts of the arteries become non-perfused (Fig. 3a. & b).

155

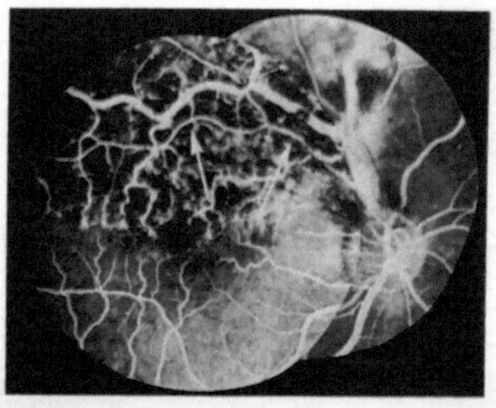

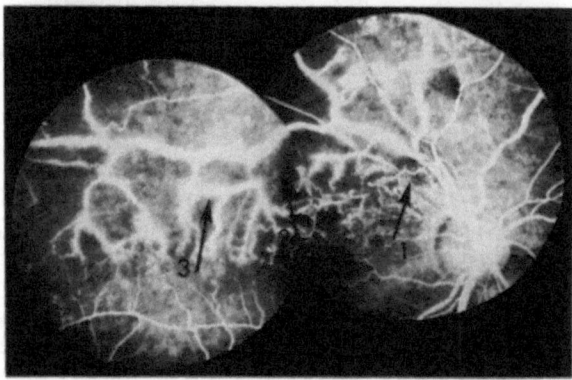

Fig. 3a. Composite picture of fluorescein angiogram of RBVO at time of first presentation, showing normal perfusion of artery (arrows).
b. Same as Fig. 3a. but 1 year later. Note narrowness and irregularity of artery near disc (arrow 1) and disappearance arterial segment (arrow 2). There is retrograde perfusion of distal segment (arrow 3).

These arteries may still be patent, as retrograde perfusion described by DOLLERY et al. (1967), is occasionally noted (Fig. 3a & b). Why arterial disease should result from vein occlusion is not immediately clear. However, when back pressure becomes high (due to outflow obstruction) arterial inflow will be reduced. This will be worsened by capillary damage and drop-out. The result will be stagnation, narrowing and eventual occlusion. The abnormal and occluded arteries observed by PATON et al. (1964), and others since, are the result and not the cause of the occlusion.

c). Capillary changes

Two types of capillary changes are observed after RBVO. In one the dominant feature is capillary dilatation, in the other capillary closure.
    In those where the main feature is capillary dilatation (this is seen when the haemorrhages have cleared) visual loss is due to macular oedema, the result of the leakage from the abnormal vessels.
    Predominant capillary closure is the common lesion in peripheral branch

156

vein occlusion. It may occur in the peri-foveal area and visual loss is then probably the result of retinal damage.

The important consequence of capillary closure is revascularisation and eventual new vessel formation (Fig. 4a & b). New vessels may also develop

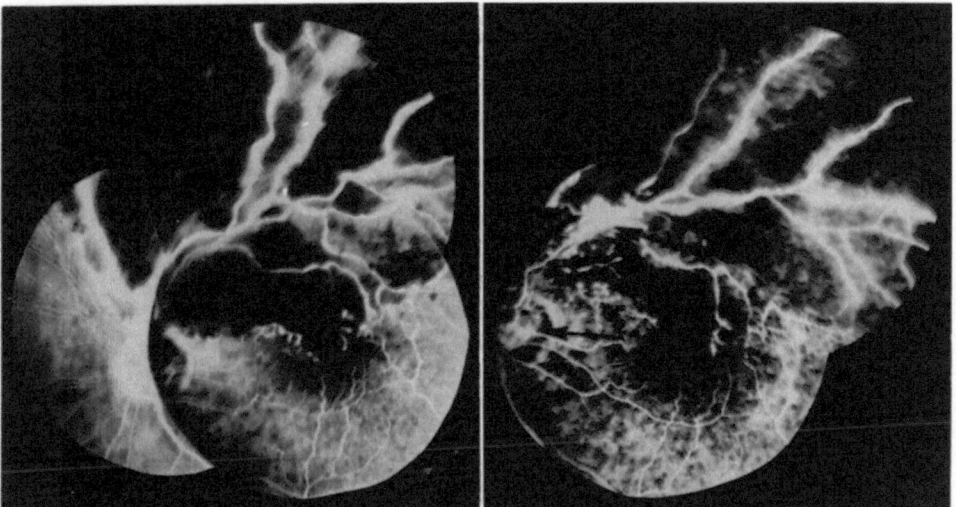

Fig. 4a. Fluorescein angiogram of RBVO in superior temporal quac rant showing large areas of capillary non-perfusion.
b. Same as Fig. 4a. but 6 months later showing new vessels de eloping along the temporal quadrant.

from the optic disc in these patients. New vessel formation ollowing RBVO has not been observed in patients who do not show large ɛ reas of capillary closure (Fig. 4a & b). Visual loss due to vitreous haemor hage from such vessels may be the presenting symptom of RBVO.

DIABETIC RETINAL VEIN OCCLUSION

1. Difference from 'classical' vein occlusion

a). Site of occlusion

In diabetic retinopathy venous abnormalities are well recognised. In the early stages functional dilatation preceding other features of retinopathy have been described (JUTTE, 1960; CAIRD et al. 1969). Later there is beading and occlusion. This can occur at any site along the vein. It almost never occurs at arterio-venous crossings and is common in the nasal retina (Fig. 5) or in the temporal periphery. The main temporal veins between the disc and macula are affected only in the most severe cases. The occlusion is thus due to primary disease of the venous wall.

157

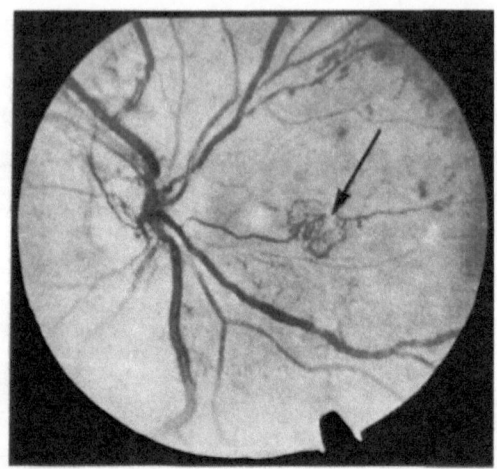

Fig. 5. From a colour transparency of L. nasal retina of diabetic patient. Arrow points at site of occlusion. Note multiple by-pass channels.

b). Capillary involvement

Capillary disease always precedes the venous occlusion of diabetes. There is always widespread capillary closure surrounding the occlusion and in the periphery. The remaining capillaries are dilated and abnormal.

c). Arterial disease

Arterial disease is frequently present as manifested by sheathing, irregularity and occlusion. Fluorescein leakage from arteries is common. In no way is the arterial disease related to the vein occlusion; it may not even be obvious in the same retinal quadrant.

2. Results of diabetic vein occlusion

By-pass channels

In diabetes the occlusion is often a gradual process, so allowing ample time for the development of collateral channels. The channels may be multiple initially and immediately by-pass the site of occlusion (Fig. 5). These multiple channels may become preretinal and take on some of the characteristics of new vessels, or may resolve into single loops. These loops may become occluded themselves if the vein reopens (Fig. 6a-c) thus emphasising that they are by-pass channels. This type of localised venous by-pass is rarely seen in the classical RBVO. This may be because the occlusion is at an arterio-venous crossing involving a major vein with few capillary tributaries rather than a small peripheral vein where capillary tributaries are frequent.

In diabetes the site of the occlusion and its collaterals are often the focus for preretinal new vessel formation, and may be attempts at revascularising

158

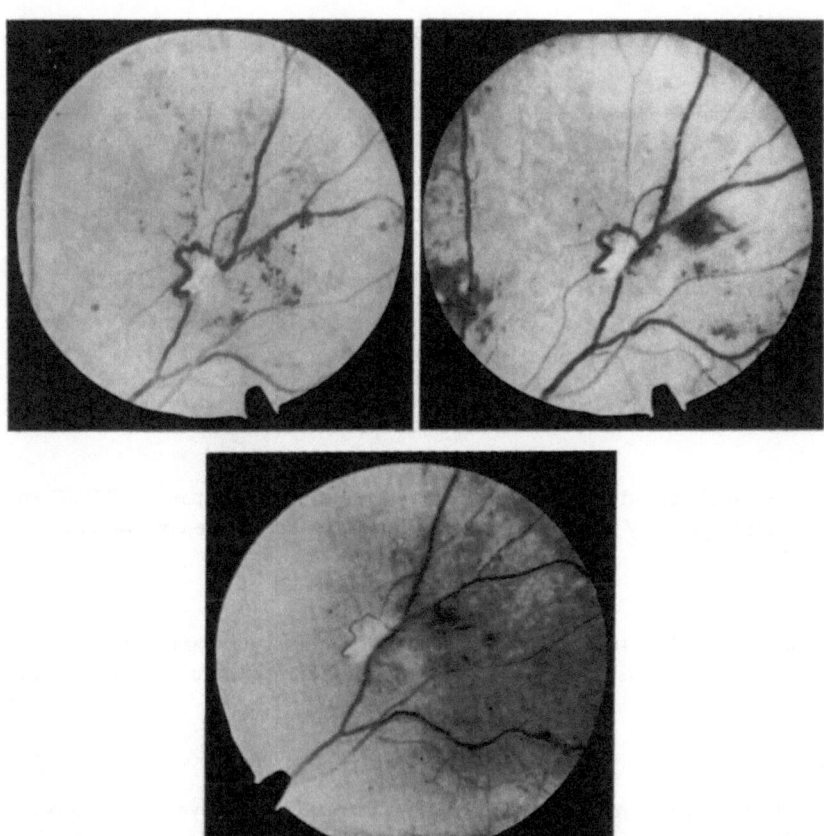

Fig. 6a. From a colour picture showing venous loop by-passing site of vein occlusion in a diabetic patient.

b. Same as Fig. 6a. but 6 months later. Note gradual disappearance of loop as vein reopens.

c. Same as Fig. 6b. but another 6 months later. Venous loop has now disappeared almost completely.

peripheral non-perfused retina. Alternatively it is possible that they are disorganized collateral channels, the result of the large areas of capillary non-perfusion.

SUMMARY AND CONCLUSIONS

It appears from the foregoing that the clinical features of RBVO are due to the obstruction of the vein. Arterial disease may be of aetiological importance, but its presence is not necessary, and in the diabetic type of vein occlusion has no relevance at all.

The two most commonly seen types of vein occlusion are similar in many of their manifestations; most important is their final outcome of new vessel formation. However, the difference between the two are more obvious and are summarized in Table I.

159

TABLE I

	Classical	Diabetic
Aetiology	Arterial disease (not occlusion)	Diabetes
Site	Arterio-venous crossing	Anywhere along vein
Capillary change	Dilatation/occlusion	Occlusion
New vessels	In those with predominant occlusion start as attempt at revascularisation	Often start as by-pass channels
Cause of visual loss	Early: macular oedema Late: vitreous haemorrhage from new vessels	– Vitreous haemorrhage from new vessels

Clear understanding of the pathogenesis and natural history of RBVO are essential before any preventive therapy or treatment can be considered.

ACKNOWLEDGMENT

We are grateful to the Consultants at Moorfields Eye Hospital for allowing us to study patients under their care. The illustrations were prepared by Mr. R. HYMPHREY.

REFERENCES

CAIRD, F.I., PIRIE, A. & RAMSELL, T.G. in: Diabetes and the Eye, p. 13, Blackwell, 1969.
CLEMETT, R.S. Brit. J. Ophthal., (1974) (in press).
DOLLERY, C.T., HILL, D.W., PATERSON, J.W. & KOHNER, E.M. Brit. J. Ophthal., 51: 249 (1967).
HAMILTON, A.M., KOHNER, E.M., ROSEN, D. & BOWBYES, J. Proc. roy. soc. Med., (1974) (in press).
HAYREH, S.S. Brit. J. Ophthal., 49: 626 (1965).
JUTTE, A. Bet. Dtch. Ophthal. Ges., 63: 419 (1960).
KOHNER, E.M., DOLLERY, C.T., PATERSON, J.W., BULPITT, C.J., HENKIND, P., SHAKIB, M. & OLIVEIRA, L. Amer. J. Ophthal., 69: 778 (1970).
KEITH, N.M., WAGENER, H.P. & BARKER, N.W. Amer. J. Med. Sci., 197: 332 (1939).
NEUBAUER, H. Bet. Dtsch. Ophthal. Ges., 63: 498 (1960).
PATON, A., RUBENSTEIN, K. & SMITH, V. Trans. Ophthal. Soc. U.K., 84: 559 (1964).
SEITZ, R. Wiener Med. Wochenschrift., 113: 180 (1963).

CLINICAL AND EPIDEMIOLOGICAL
ASSOCIATION OF RETINAL VEIN OCCLUSION
AND CEREBRAL STROKE

S. MERIN & L. YANKO

(Jerusalem, Israel)

The classical picture of ipsilateral blindness and contralateral paralysis due to carotid and ophthalmic artery occlusion is well known to ophthalmologists. It is less known that retinal vein thrombosis is much more frequently associated with cerebral stroke than chance would allow. The following four patients seen by us in the last two years illustrate the clinical association between these two findings. I would like to describe them briefly.

The first patient was a 60 year old slightly hypertensive man who suffered a sudden loss of vision in his right eye. The eye examination revealed a central retinal vein thrombosis in this eye and many A/V crossing pressure signs in the left eye. No treatment was suggested. Three weeks later a sudden left hemiparesis appeared, including weakness of the left part of the face and the left upper and lower extremity.

The second patient was a 61-year old hypertensive man who suffered a sudden loss of vision in his left eye. On the same night he felt a dizziness and his whole right side including the face became paralyzed. An eye examination revealed a central vein thrombosis. The general examination did not show any remarkable findings except a blood pressure of 200/135. He recovered from the paralysis but one and a half year later a second cerebro-vascular accident in form of a right hemiparesis with aphasia occured. In the left eye a hemorrhagic glaucoma turned the eye to be blind and painful which necessitated its enucleation.

The retina showed extensive destruction and gliosis. A transverse section of the optic nerve at the 1.5 mm' level revealed hypertrophy of the media of the central retinal artery while at the 2.5 mm' level a coagulum is seen which occludes the lumen of the central retinal vein.

The third patient was a 58-year old woman who suffered a right upper temporal branch vein thrombosis. The general examination revealed a high blood pressure of 210/110. A year later she suffered from a mild left hemiparesis. Ophthalmodynamometric measurements at that time revealed a significant difference between the diastolic pressure of two eyes: 80 mm Hg in the right and 100 in the left.

The fourth patient was a 48-year old hypertensive woman, suffering from chronic schizophrenia. An eye examination, done because of visual complaints revealed a severe hypertensive retinopathy and a central retinal vein thrombosis in the right eye. In addition a left hemiparesis was found.

Ophthalmodynamometric values were significantly different between the two eyes, the diastolic pressure being 50 mm' in the right eye and 80 mm' in the left eye.

Let us now turn to the literature. FOSTER MOORE (1924) found that during 8 years, 15 out of 36 patients with central retinal vein thrombosis developed a cerebral stroke. This means that 41% of his patients followed for 8 years had the association which is the topic of this paper.

LOWE & STEPHENS (1961) when studying ophthalmodynamometry during carotid artery compression found that they had one complication: an elderly hypertensive patient developed a retinal vein thrombosis.

A clinical resemblance to retinal vein occlusion is found in a series of conditions known to be associated with carotid artery decreased blood flow, as in occlusion of the carotid artery or its artificial ligation (DOWLING & SMITH, 1960; HOLLENHORST, 1962), including the condition described as venous stasis retinopathy (KEARNS & HOLLENHORST, 1963).

Fluorescein angiography which typically shows a delay in vessel filling in cases of vein occlusion shows a similar delay in carotid compression, carotid ligation or carotid occlusion (DAVID et al., 1966; LAVENSTEIN et al., 1971; WINKELMAN et al., 1971).

In summary, the combination of clinical cases such as these described here, epidemiological studies such as the one by FOSTER MOORE and some established clinical facts about the retinopathy and retinal vessel filling in cases of carotid artery occlusion indicate that the association of retinal vein thrombosis and cerebral stroke is not a fortuitous one.

REFERENCES

DAVID, N.J., NORTON, E.W.D., GASS, J.D.M. & SEXTON, R. Fluorescein retinal angiography in carotid occlusion. *Arch. Neurol.*, 14: *281-287* (1966).

DOWLING, J.L. & SMITH, T.R. An ocular study of pulseless disease. *Arch. Ophthal.*, 64: *236-242* (1960).

HOLLENHORST, R.W. Carotid and vertebral-basilar arterial stenosis and occlusion; neuro-ophthalmologic considerations. *Trans. Amer. Acad. Ophthal. & Otol.*, 66: *166-180* (1962).

KEARNS, T.P. & HOLLENHORST, R.W. Venous-stasis retinopathy of occlusive disease of the carotid artery. *Proc. Mayo Clin.*, 38: *304-312* (1963).

LAVENSTEIN, B., MILDER, B., WINKELMAN, J.Z., ZAPPIA, R.J. & GAY, A.J. Retinal and choroidal circulation in rabbits. *Arch. Ophthal.*, 85: *723* (1971).

LOWE, R.D. & STEPHENS, N.L. Carotid occlusion. Its diagnosis by ophthalmodynamometry during carotid compression. *Lancet* I: *1241-1245* (1961).

MOORE, R.F. Retinal venous thrombosis. A clinical study of sixty-two cases followed over many years. *Brit. J. Ophthal.*, Suppl. 2 (1924).

WINKELMAN, J.Z., ZAPPIA, R.J. & GAY, A.J. Human arm to retina circulation time. *Arch. Ophthal.*, 86: *626-636* (1971).

TREATMENT OF VENOUS STASIS
RETINOPATHY
A PRELIMINARY REPORT

SOHAN SINGH HAYREH

(Iowa City, Iowa)

In the treatment of central retinal vein occlusion a wide variety of therapeutic regimens have been tried from time to time. These include anticoagulants, fibrinolytic agents, low molecular weight Dextran infusion, chlorifibrate, photocoagulation, retrobular injection of steroids, vasodilators or alphachymotrypsin. Of all these agents, anticoagulants have been the most commonly used (PLOMAN, 1938; HOLMIN & PLOMAN, 1938; MACDONALD, 1940, 1951; LARSSON & NORD, 1950; DUFF et al., 1951; KLIEN & OLWIN, 1956; MYLIUS & WITT, 1957; GLEES, 1959; WITMER, 1959) with some claiming varying degrees of success while others feel it makes no significant difference in the outcome of visual acuity as compared to the untreated cases (LARSON & NORD, 1950; GLEES, 1959; LISTER & ZWINK, 1953; TIBURTIUS, 1960).

I feel the basis of most of the conflicting claims for various treatments could be partly due to our ignorance of the natural history of the disease, and partly to the fact that cases of venous stasis retinopathy and haemorrhagic retinopathy are included together as so-called central retinal vein occlusion, when, in fact, the two conditions are not identical (HAYREH, 1974). A review of most of the reports indicates a high success rate with various treatments in cases where the description suggests that the patients were suffering from venous stasis retinopathy; the poorest outcome was in cases with haemorrhagic retinopathy. I have described elsewhere the pathogenesis of venous stasis retinopathy and the differentiating features between venous stasis retinopathy and haemorrhagic retinopathy (HAYREH, 1974). Although venous stasis retinopathy is a benign and self-limited condition, resolving in about a couple of years and may not significantly impair the visual acuity; in some cases it does produce macular oedema which not only lowers the visual acuity but also may result in cystoid macular degeneration and permanent central scotoma. Thus, treatment in venous stasis retinopathy consists of resolving the macular oedema to retain the central vision. Recently I have treated some of these cases with systemic corticosteroids which have given encouraging results.

The prevalent concept that these venous stasis retinopathy cases represent partial, incipient, or impending central retinal vein occlusion and that anticoagulants should prevent them from going on to a complete occlusion is not correct because a vast majority of these never progress to haemorrhagic retinopathy in spite of no treatment. In the present series none showed such a progression.

MATERIAL AND METHODS

Twenty-eight patients with venous stasis retinopathy were studied. They had complete ocular and systemic examinations, including recording of visual fields, stereoscopic colour fundus photography and intravenous fluorescein fundus angiography. These patients were followed-up at regular intervals by recording visual acuity, ophthalmoscopic appearances, visual fields, and, on some occasions, fluorescein fundus angiography. Fourteen of these patients were put on systemic corticosteroids with 40-60 mgm prednisolone as a starting daily dose and then gradually tapered, with visual acuity as the main criterion in regulation of the dosage. The remaining 14 patients had no treatment but were followed similar to the treated group. The results of this study were submitted to statistical analysis by using Fisher's Exact Test to determine statistical significance of the results.

OBSERVATIONS AND COMMENTS

Age:

These patients usually fall into two groups, i.e., young adults and the old age group. I have used 50 years as the arbitrary dividing line between these two age groups. Based on this, the age incidence in this series was as follows:
A. Young group: This included 9 patients belonging to an age group of 23 to 49 (35 *b* 8.7) years.
B. Old group: In this group there were 19 patients within the ages of 52 to 77 (61 *b* 7.5) years.

I feel, based on these and previous observations, (1971) that venous stasis retinopathy can occur in young adults as well as in old age, although comparatively more frequently in the latter. In the young adults the venous stasis retinopathy is without any associated vascular sclerosis and the primary cause in all probability is phlebitis of the central retinal vein in the region of the optic nerve head or retrolaminar region; this leads to localized thrombosis of the vein.

In the old age group, the primary cause is thought to be arteriosclerosis, producing compression, secondary epithelial proliferation and thrombosis of the central retinal vein in the optic nerve (KLIEN & OLWIN, 1956; KLIEN, 1966). This difference in the pathogenesis of venous stasis retinopathy in the young and old may have some bearing on our management of the condition in the two groups, e.g. corticosteroids would be indicated in the young group to control the inflammatory process.

Sex:

There were 22 (78%) males and 6 (22%) females in this series. The incidence of sex distribution in the young and old groups was as follows:

A. Young group:	Males	— 6 (21%)
	Females	— 3 (11%)
B. Old group:	Males	— 16 (57%)
	Females	— 3 (11%)

This suggest that venous stasis retinopathy is more commonly seen in males (78%), than females (22%) and this difference in sex distribution was statistically very significant (P < 0.01).

Side:

Venous stasis retinopathy involved the left side much more frequently than the right side, as is evident from Table I and this difference in the

TABLE I

Age group	Sex	Side (Number of eyes with % incidence)		
		Left eye	Right eye	Bilateral
Young	Male	4 (14%)	1 (3.5%)	*1 (3.5%)
	Female	2 (7%)	1 (3.5%)	–
Old	Male	10 (36%)	6 (21.5%)	–
	Female	3 (11%)	–	–
Overall		19 (68%)	8 (28.5%)	1 (3.5%)

*Left eye involved 3 1/4 years before the right eye.

distribution between the two eyes was statistically significant (P < 0.05).

In this series there was only one case where the right eye was involved 3 1/4 years after the involvement of the left eye in a young male. Since the follow-up period in the present series is less than three years, it is possible that this series does not reflect a true incidence of bilateral disease. A similar involvement of the second eye 2 1/2 years after the involvement of the first eye has been brought to my attention by MUNRO (HAYREH, 1971).

No satisfactory explanation is available for the statistically significant high preponderance of venous stasis retinopathy in males (78%) and on the left side (68%).

Follow-up period:

These patients were followed-up for 5 to 34 (17 ±9) months, with bilateral venous stasis retinopathy in one patient having been followed in retrospect for 14 1/2 years (by me for two years). Four of these patients are still being followed on treatment.

Interval between the onset of visual disturbance and first ophthalmic consultation:

I.   Found on a routine ophthalmoscopic examination,
      with no visual complaint   = 5 patients
II.   One day or less   = 3 patients
III. Four to five days   = 2 patients
IV.   One to eight (4 ± 2.5) weeks   = 16 patients
V.   Sixteen to 24 weeks   = 2 patients
Initial presenting symptoms:

165

I.	No complaint	= 5 patients
II.	Intermittent transient blurring of vision lasting from a few seconds to a few hours (in 6 patients the blurring was worse in the morning)	= 12 patients
III.	Blurred vision of gradual onset	= 6 patients
IV.	Blurred vision of sudden onset	= 5 patients

Initial visual acuity:

Table II summarizes the visual acuity at the time of first consultation. This

TABLE II

Initial Visual Acuity in 29 Eyes

Visual acuity	6/6 or better	6/7.5- 6/9	6/12- 6/15	6/18	6/24	6/36	6/60	C.F.*
Inci- dence	38%	38%	14%	–	3.5%	3.5%	–	3.5%

*Counts fingers

table is significant because it shows that visual acuity in these cases is in no way nearly as bad as in haemorrhagic retinopathy. It is more often the annoyance and apprehension caused by the blurred central vision then the severity of the visual loss that brings the patient for consultation. Only three out of 29 eyes had a visual acuity or less than 6/12 - 6/15.

Corticosteroid therapy:

An attempt has been made to evaluate the role of steroid therapy in venous stasis retinopathy.

1. Patient selection

The patient had to have had venous stasis retinopathy and a significantly poor visual acuity to qualify for corticosteroid therapy.

In addition young persons were treated because of the possibility of venous stasis retinopathy being secondary to phlebitis (p. 4).

a. Diagnosis of venous stasis retinopathy:

This was made on a combination of history, visual acuity, visual field defects, and ophthalmoscopic and fluorescein angiographic appearances (HAYREH, 1974). There is history of blurred vision, mainly in the central field, which is frequently worse in the morning and gradually gets better as the day passes. The visual acuity in 76% is 6/9 or better (or in 90% 6/12 or better). The peripheral visual fields with very small targets are normal or near normal, and the main defect which is present involves usually the central field, i.e., a central scotoma or distortion, best outlined on an

166

Amsler grid chart. On ophthalmoscopy the retinal veins are markedly engorged and tortuous, with or without retinal haemorrhages, which vary from a new flame-shaped and punctate types to a large number in the central part and usually more frequent punctate haemorrhages in the peripheral part of the fundus; however, these haemorrhages are almost always much less extensive than those seen in haemorrhagic retinopathy. The optic disc shows hyperaemia and usually certain amount of oedema. In late cases the disc usually shows the presence of retinociliary veins. Cotton-wool spots are rare and seen only in severe cases. The macular region may be normal, have a few haemorrhages or may show oedema; presence of a central foveal haemorrhage may sometimes be seen, leading to markedly poor visual acuity. Fluorescein angiography shows a marked venous stasis with or without dilated retinal capillaries and/or microaneurysms, no obliteration of retinal capillaries, no retinal neovascularization, leakage of fluorescein along the main retinal veins and their tributaries (maximum along the main veins, with maximim pooling in the concavities of the big veins), the optic disc and the macula (in cases with macular oedema) and there may be late fluorescein staining of the retina.

b. Visual acuity:

For consideration of corticosteroid therapy the venous stasis retinopathy patients could be divided into the following three groups on the basis of their visual acuity.

Group I: In this group there were ten eyes (nine old and one young) which showed no significant drop in visual acuity and required no treatment. Three of these eyes were discovered to have venous stasis retinopathy on a routine ophthalmic examination. In this group, although the majority had a mild fluctuation in visual acuity or complained of blurred vision, objective testing revealed a normal visual acuity.

Group II: This consisted of five eyes (4 patients) where the visual acuity deteriorated significantly but no therapy was given because of either systemic contraindications or the ophthalmologist in charge did not agree to this therapy. In this group three eyes (2 patients) were of the young age group and two of the old age group.

Group III: This was the treated group. Fourteen eyes belonged to this group (five young and nine old persons). The decision to start systemic corticosteroids was made only after the eyes developed a significant drop in their visual acuity and showed evidence of macular oedema on ophthalmoscopy and/or fluorescein angiography. The visual acuity at the start of therapy in this group was as follows (Table III):

A comparison of the visual acuities in Table III with those in Table II clearly demonstrates a very significant ($P < 0.001$) fall of visual acuity in these cases before a decision to treat them with corticosteroids was taken.

This poor visual acuity developed at the following time intervals after the onset of visual symptoms:

I. Simultaneous with the onset of visual symptoms   = 5 eyes
II. About a month or two after onset of visual
    symptoms   = 5 eyes

III.   About 6 months after onset of visual symptoms   = 9 eyes

If the visual acuity dropped simultaneously with the onset of symptoms, it could be that the venous stasis retinopathy was symptomless to begin with and the development of macular oedema produced deterioration of visual acuity. Occasionally it was due to a foveal haemorrhage.

TABLE III

Visual Acuity at the Start of Steroid Therapy in 14 Eyes

Visual acuity	6/6 or better	6/7.5- 6/9	6/12- 6/15	6/18	6/24	6/36	6/60	C.F.*
Inci- dence	38%	7%	14%	28%	14%	14%	14%	7%

*Counts fingers

2. Dosage

The patients were given 40-60 mgm of oral prednisone or prednisolone per day in divided doses. Higher doses were given in patients with severe venous stasis retinopathy and comparatively marked deterioration of vision. The patients felt a dramatic subjective visual improvement within a day or two of the start of therapy and usually a significant improvement of the visual acuity objectively but no change in ophthalmoscopic appearances of the fundus. Once the vision started to improve, the patient was advised to continuously and slowly decrease the dose of prednisone to a level which prevented deterioration of vision. Each patient was titrated slowly for the dosage corresponding with his visual acuity. The objective was to work out the lowest possible symptom-free maintenance dose. If a deterioration developed during the process of reduction, dose was increased to produce an improvement. It was discovered that there was a certain level of dosage below which steroids produced no improvement initially and the vision showed signs of deterioration. It is something like an 'all-or-none law' response. In the present series this minimum required dose was usually 40 mgm of prednisone daily. If these patients were given a dose less than that, they showed none or no significant improvement but once given the adequate dose there was a good response. This fact is extremely important because timidly giving inadequate amounts of steroids would serve no useful purpose other than to bring discredit to this treatment. I have found that if on tapering off or on stopping steroids, visual deterioration occurs, one must start once again with the highest dose which originally produced an improvement; small inadequate doses will usually produce no improvement. The maximum dose and the maintenance dose required for improvement vary from person to person and no generalization can be made. Some patients may have to be given an initial dose of as high as 80 mgm or even more to produce a good response, gradually tapering this to a maintenance dose.

168

3. Duration

Steroid therapy in these cases had to be continued for months because of the chronic nature of venous stasis retinopathy. The objective of treatment is usually not to treat venous stasis retinopathy (which is a self-limited condition and we have as yet no satisfactory treatment for this disease), but to keep the macular oedema under control and thus prevent development of cystoid macular degeneration and permanent loss of central vision. In young adults where venous stasis retinopathy is supposed to be inflammatory in origin, steroids may be helpful to treat the retinopathy itself. In the present series the duration of the treatment was as follows:
I. In four cases tapering off of the steroids, when the visual acuity had returned to normal, produced no recurrence or deterioration of vision. The required treatment for a period of 9, 10, 12 and 20 weeks.
II. In some of the remaining ten patients, reduction of prednisolone below about 40 mgm (in a few 20-30 mgm) resulted in deterioration of vision. Whenever the steroids were increased to adequate dosage, the visual acuity improved but again deteriorated on reduction. Frequently, although the visual acuity was not maintained at the best level on low dosage, it was better than that without any treatment. After it was established in each case that the steroids helped, they were often given the following three options.
a. Either to take a dose big enough to remain symptomfree and with a satisfactory visual acuity but suffer from some of the side-effects of this therapy since this therapy may have to be continued longer than a year or so;
b. Or to take a smaller dose as a compromise between lower visual acuity but less chance of developing side-effects from steroid therapy;
c. Or having no therapy at all and be willing to take a high risk of losing central vision.
   In this group the treatment was given for a period varying from two weeks to about a year and four patients are still on a maintenance dose of 15 mgm (in 2) and 30 mgm (in 2) daily after 12, 9, 4 and 4 1/2 months respectively. In the remaining six patients the steroids were stopped either because of development of side-effects or in view of associated systemic diseases or the patient took the option (c). In all except one of these patients visual acuity dropped to 6/24 to 6/60; in one normal visual acuity was finally recovered.

4. Evaluation

The primary criterion used for evaluation of the effectivity of steroid therapy was the visual acuity; in addition, the Amsler grid chart and in some cases central visual fields, if the latter showed any defect, were also used to assess the therapy. It must be stressed strongly that ophthalmoscopic appearance cannot be used for such an evaluation because, over a short period of time, these show no significant change in spite of a marked improvement in the visual acuity. Thus absence of improvement in ophthalmoscopic appearances is no criterion that the steroid therapy is not effective. It takes weeks or months for a significant change to be evident in

169

the fundus picture, whereas visual acuity improvement is seen within 2 - 3 days or so.

Since all the 14 patients in Group III did not take any therapy throughout the period of defective vision and follow-up and to begin with they were put on therapy only when they showed a significant deterioration in visual acuity, the initial and final visual acuities of this treated group (14 patients of Group III − p. 10) cannot be compared with those of the untreated group (14 patients of Groups I and II − p. 10) to evaluate the beneficial effect of steroid therapy in venous stasis retinopathy. Only the group II (p. 10) can be considered comparable with the Group III (p. 10) for this purpose. Another very important parameter can be used to evaluate the effectivity of steroid therapy in each patient within Group III itself, i.e., a comparison of visual acuities just before the start of therapy, at an adequate dosage level, after withdrawal of therapy and at the end of follow-up (Table IV and Fig. 1). There was a distinct improvement on adequate corticosteroid therapy. A visual acuity of 6/12 or better was seen in only 21% before the therapy, but was seen in 91% with adequate dosage. On comparing the visual acuities at the start of the therapy with that of the adequate steroid therapy, the improvement in visual acuity to 6/12 or better with therapy was very highly significant ($P < 0.001$). In the untreated five eyes of Group II (p. 10) no significant ($P < 0.5$) difference was detected between the initial and final visual acuities. This establishes the beneficial effect of steroid therapy in these cases.

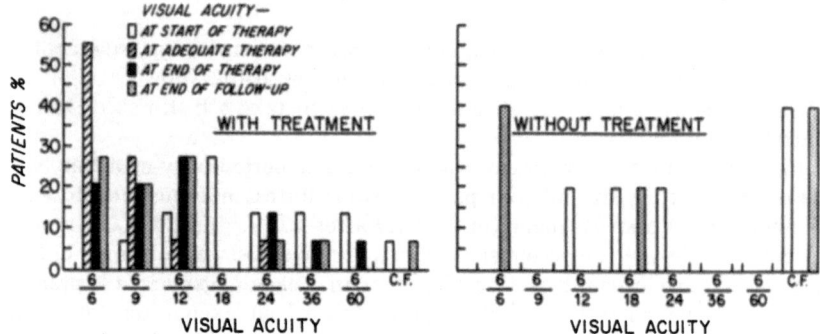

Fig. 1. Graphic representation of the visual acuities in treated (Group III) and untreated (Group II) cases at different stages. Abscissa shows the visual acuities and ordinate the incidende in percentage in the eyes.

The results of the untreated eyes in Group II suggest that these eyes ultimately either recover normal visual acuity (in 2 eyes) or end up with a central scotoma (in 3 eyes − visual acuity of counts fingers in 2 and 6/18 in one).

Table V summarizes a further analysis of the response to treatment by the young as compared to the old age group. On comparing the visual acuity at the start of the therapy with that at the adequate steroid therapy, the improvement in visual acuity to 6/9 or better was much more significant in the old group ($P < 0.01$) than the young group ($P < 0.05$). This may be

TABLE IV

Visual Acuity and Therapy

	In treated cases (Group III)				In untreated cases (Group II)	
	V.A. at start of Rx	V.A. at adequate dose	V.A. at end of Rx	Final V.A.	Initial	Final
6/6 or better	–	56%	21%	28%	–	40%
6/7.5-6/9	7%	28%	21%	21%	–	–
6/12-6/15	14%	7%	28%	28%	20%	20%
6/18	28%	–	–	–	20%	–
6/24	14%	7%	14%	7%	20%	–
6/36	14%	–	7%	7%	–	–
6/60	14%	–	7%	–	–	–
C.F.*	7%	–	–	7%	40%	40%

CF. * = counts fingers

partly due to the fact that the initial visual acuity in the old group was much worse than the young group. However, no statistically significant difference was detected in the visual acuities at different stages in Table V between the young and the old.

TABLE V

Visual Acuity, Age and Treatment

| | Treated Group | | | | | |
| | V.A. at start of Rx | | V.A. with adequate Rx | | Final V.A. | |
	Young	Old	Young	Old	Young	Old
6/6	–	–	60%	55%	40%	22%
6/9	20%	–	40%	22%	20%	22%
6/12	20%	11%	–	11%	40%	22%
6/18	20%	33%	–	–	–	–
6/24	20%	11%	–	11%	–	11%
6/36	20%	11%	–	–	–	11%
6/60	–	22%	–	–	–	11%
C.F.*	–	11%	–	–	–	–
No of eyes	5	9				

*C.F. = counts fingers

5. Retinociliary veins:

These were seen in 21 out of 29 eyes of this series. It was difficult to determine the exact time interval between the onset of venous stasis retinopathy and the development of retinociliary veins, mainly because exact time of onset of the venous stasis retinopathy was not definite. The onset of visual symptoms in venous stasis retinopathy does not necessarily coincide with the onset of the retinopathy because in five cases the retinopathy was first detected on a routine ophthalmic examination with no visual symptoms whatsoever and in one of these retinociliary veins were already present. In five eyes the retinociliary veins were seen on first consulation although the symptoms were present only for one week to two months. Thus in 9 out of 29 eyes it was impossible to determine the time of onset of the occlusion. With this big reservation in mind, the approximate time interval between the onset of venous stasis retinopathy and development of retinociliary veins can be six months or so. In eight eyes no retinociliary veins were seen and these eyes were followed from eight months to a year (with one followed for 28 months). No relationship was seen between the presence or absence of retinociliary veins and the visual acuity on therapy or otherwise.

6. Systemic diseases:

In this series 15 patients had the following one or more systemic diseases

Arterial hypertension	=	6 patients
Diabetes + arterial hypertension	=	2 patients
Diabetes	=	1 patient
Carotid artery stenosis	=	2 patients
Peripheral vascular disease	=	2 patients
Last trimester of pregnancy	=	1 patient
On high doses of oestrogen for menopausal syndrome	=	1 patient
Peptic ulcer history	=	3 patients
History of past pulmonary tuberculosis	=	1 patient

In some of these patients these systemic conditions either contra-indicated steroid therapy or indicated a guarded administration with minimal dose and short duration in spite of a satisfactory response and normal visual acuity with adequate dosage. Thus, systemic diseases may limit the administration of adequate dosage and its duration to safeguard the macula against macular degeneration.

7. Other therapies

a. In the patient with bilateral venous stasis retinopathy, the retinopathy in the first eye, with a visual acuity of 6/6, was treated with anticoagulants by the ophthalmologist in charge; this produced vitreous haemorrhage (the only eye in this series with vitreous haemorrhage) and the patient was left with a macular degeneration and counts fingers vision. When he developed venous stasis retinopathy in the second eye, no therapy of any kind was given and he recovered a visual acuity of 6/6 after an initial fall of visual acuity to 6/18.
b. In one patient, aspirin was given as an initial therapy. Within three weeks his visual acuity deteriorated to 6/15 from 6/6. On putting him on systemic steroids his visual acuity returned to normal in three weeks.

These two case reports are mentioned simply as observations, with no definite conclusions.

Limitations of this study:

It may rightly be argued that this study has the following limitations:
1. It is not a randomized double-blind controlled study.
2. There is no adequate control group to compare the results of the treated group.

While I fully accept these limitations, I would like to point out that in this treated group there was a certain amount of individual control observed. This control has been the presence of a direct relationship between the administration of adequate amounts of steroids and improvement in visual acuity, i.e., adequate doses of steroids improved the visual acuity immediately, withdrawal of steroids produced marked deterioration of vision and once again administration of adequate steroids resulted in good visual acuity (Fig. 2). This indicates that in spite of the above mentioned objections, this study does indicate a definite beneficial effect by systemic steroids on the visual acuity in venous stasis retinopathy. However, it does not give us any

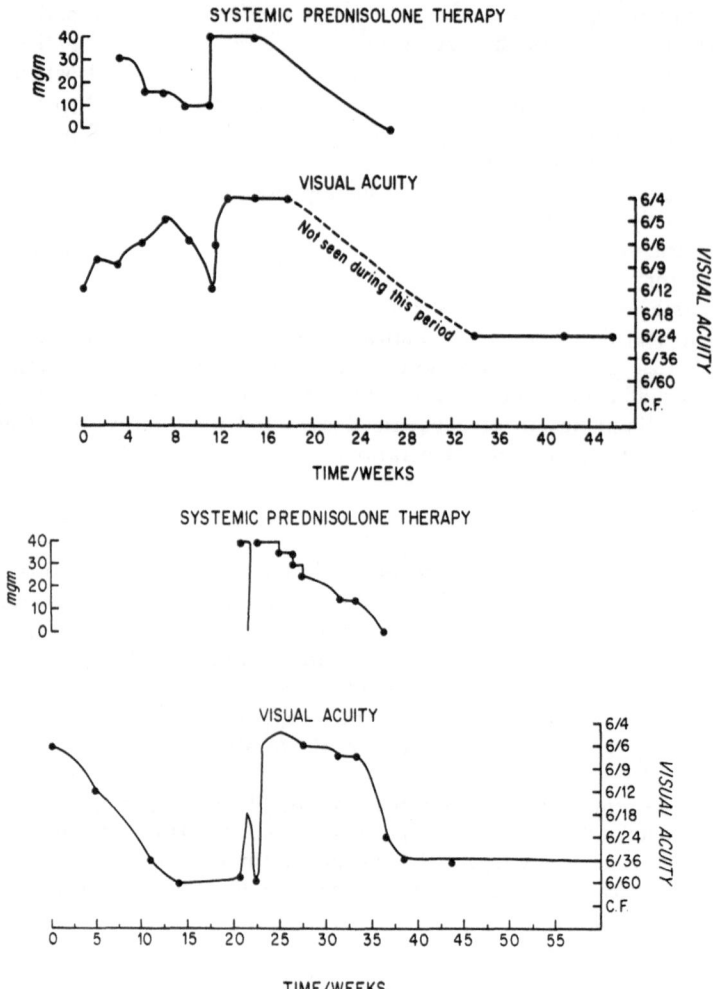

Fig. 2. Graphic representation of the response of visual acuity to oral prednisolone tablets in (a) 61-year-old man and (b) 64-year-old woman.

In both patients the steroid therapy was stopped because of development of side-effects of steroid therapy.

information as to whether the steroid therapy shortens the course of the disease. In the young group, there is some evidence that adequate steroid therapy significantly reduces the course and complications of venous stasis retinopathy.

Based on the encouraging results by this preliminary study, I propose to do a large and long-term randomized double-blind controlled study on the subject.

Administration of subtenon's steroids to replace the systemic therapy has been suggested to avoid the systemic side-effects of steroid therapy. I have not tried this method so far because of its uncertain effectivity combined

174

with the discomfort of repeated, somewhat painful, injections over a period of months or even longer.

Choices open for a patient with venous stasis retinopathy associated with significantly deteriorated central vision

There are mainly two choices open to such a patient:
1. To have long-term systemic steroid therapy lasting for months or even longer with very high chances of retention of good vision but run the risk of suffering from side-effects of such a therapy;
2. To have no treatment and run a high risk of permanent loss of central vision. I must add here that there were persons in this series who recovered normal vision in spite of no treatment, as was the case in three patients with initial visual acuities of about 6/18, although this was uncommon.

This would naturally confront the patients as well as the ophthalmologist with a dilemma. Both options carry certain amounts of risk and the decision would rest upon multiple factors. In patients with venous stasis retinopathy but no significant fall of visual acuity, no treatment is indicated except for a close watch on their visual acuity and the fundus appearances.

SUMMARY AND CONCLUSIONS

Venous stasis retinopathy is a self-limited, chronic and comparatively benign condition as compared to haemorrhagic retinopathy. The main complication which requires management is the deterioration of central visual acuity ultimately resulting in a central scotoma due to development of macular oedema and, if untreated, ending in cystoid macular degeneration. Thus the indication for treatment in these cases is the fall of central visual acuity of the 29 eyes (28 patients) with venous stasis retinopathy in the present series, 10 eyes showed no deterioration of vision throughout the entire course of follow-up (Group I) and hence required no treatment. The remaining 19 eyes developed deterioration of vision; five eyes (four patients) amongst these were not treated in spite of the disturbance of vision (Group II) while the other 14 eyes (Group III) were treated by systemic corticosteroids starting with a dose of 40-60 mgm of oral prednisolone daily and then gradually tapering off to a maintenance dose. Results of Group III cases strongly suggested that adequate doses of systemic steroids help to prevent deterioration of vision and in recovery of deteriorated vision; possibly without altering significantly the course of venous stasis retinopathy itself. However, they require long-term therapy for months or even longer during the course of venous stasis retinopathy because on stopping the therapy poor visual acuity recurred in 10 of these eyes. This factor may limit the usefulness of this therapy if contraindications to such prolonged steroid therapy or side effects of steroid therapy exist in a patient. In such cases one may be confronted with the dilemma of either not to treat these cases and run a fairly high risk of permanent loss of central vision, or treating them with adequate doses of systemic steroids, retaining good visual acuity but running the risk of side-effects from prolonged steroid therapy. The decision under such circumstances may not be easy but this study had indicated the beneficial·effects from adequate doses of steroid therapy in such cases, many of whom otherwise would end up with a central scotoma.

While evaluating the effectivity of steroid therapy, improvement in visual acuity should be the primary criterion becauce the fundus appearances almost always show no significant improvement for weeks in spite of the visual acuity rapidly returning to a normal level.

ACKNOWLEDGEMENTS

I owe a debt of gratitude to many ophthalmologists for referring these patients to me, to DR E.B. FRENCH of the University of Edinburgh and to the Cardio-Vascular Unit of the University of Iowa for systemic evaluation of these patients, and to MR L. BURMEISTER of the Biostatistic Department, University of Iowa for statistical analysis of the results, and to MRS. MARIA WARBASSE for her secretarial assistance.

REFERENCES

DUFF I.F.,FALLS H.F. & LINMAN, J.W. Anticoagulant therapy in occlusive vascular disease of the retina. *Arch. Ophthal. (Chicago)*, 46: s,601 (1951).

GLEES, M. Ueber Erfahrungen mit Thrombozid bei der Zentralvenenthrombose. *Klin. Mbl. Augenheilk.* 134: *807* (1959).

HAYREH, S.S. Pathogenesis of occlusion of the central retinal vessels. *Amer. J. Ophthal.* 72: *998* (1971).

HAYREH S.S. Optic disc vasculitis. *Brit. J, Ophthal.* 56: *625* (1972).

HAYREH S.S. Central retinal vascular occlusion: Morphology and Pathogenesis. Proc. IX Intern. Cong. Angiology, Florence, 1974, Minerva Cardioangiol. (In press).

HAYREH S.S. Pathogenesis of central retinal vein occlusion.

HOLMIN, N. & PLOMAN K.G. Thrombosis of central vein of retina treated with heparin. *Lancet* 1: *664* (1938).

KLIEN, B.A. & OLWIN J.H. A survey of the pathogenesis of retinal venous occlusion. *Arch. Ophthal.* (Chicago) 56: *207* (1956).

KLIEN, B.A. Sidelights on retinal venous occlusion. *Amer. J. Ophthal.* 61: *25* (1966).

LARSSON, S. & NORD, B. Some remarks on retinal vein thrombosis and its treatment with anticoagulants. *Acta Ophthal. (Kbh.)*, 28: *187* (1950).

LISTER, A. & ZWINK F.B. The course of thrombosis of the retinal veins. *Trans. ophthal.Soc. U.K.* 73: *55* (1953).

MACDONALD A.E. Heparin in thrombosis of the central vein. *Trans. Amer. ophthal. Soc.* 38: *313* (1940).

MACDONALD A.E. In discussion. *Arch. Ophthal.(Chicago)*, 46: *615* (1951).

MYLIUS, K. & WITT, G. Ueber die Behandlung der Netzhautvenenthrombose mit Thrombocid. *Klin. Mbl. Augenheilk.* 131: 145 (1957).

PLOMAN, K.G. Treatment of thrombosis of the veins of the retina with Heparin. *Acta Ophthal. (Kbh.)* 16: *502* (1938).

TIBURTIUS H. Ueber Venenverschlusse der Netzhaut. *Klin. Mbl. Augenheilk.* 136: *604* (1960).

WITMER, R. Zur Behandlung der Retina-Venenthrombosen. *Klin. Mbl. Augenheilk.* 134: *797* (1959).

HOME EYE TEST

VIRGINIA S. BOYCE*

(New York, U.S.A.)

The National Society's recommendation is that every child should have an eye examination at birth and then again before entering school. This is an ideal that probably will not be realized for many years. One in every 20 preschool aged children is affected by a vision problem, the most serious being amblyopia. This condition can usually be corrected if discovered and treatment initiated before the age of six or seven years. Early detection, therefore, is crucial. Our efforts have been directed at training volunteers to conduct community preschool vision screening programs. So far we have been able to reach only some 500,000 prescholers each year while our potential audience is 15,000,000 children between the ages 3 and 6.

In our search for an answer to close this gap we learned of a screening test designed to be administered at home by the parent. This was conceived by the Sight Conservation Research Center of San Jose, California. Four important questions needed answers:

1. Could the screening techniques involved in these tests be communicated to parents?
2. Could parents in turn secure the cooperation and comprehension of children at such an early age?
3. Would parents accept the fact that their child could not pass the test and take him or her to the doctor?
4. Was the test valid and reliable?

For three years the local ophthalmological community and the National Society's Committee on Eye Health of Children conducted evaluations with these points in mind. The findings were positive in all respects and results were judged comparable to the traditional community screening. Reinforcing this view was the experience reported from several other areas where similar testing was underway.

It appeared that we finally had a device for reaching children nationwide, whether in remote rural areas or in what has become known as the inner city.

To eliminate the chance that the test might be misunderstood and contribute to a false sense of security, we stressed in our publicity, and in the test kit itself, that the Home Eye Test is not diagnostic and should in no way take the place of a complete eye examination. It was further emphasized that this is a simple screening test for distance visual acuity and

*Executive Director, National Society for the Prevention of Blindness, Inc.

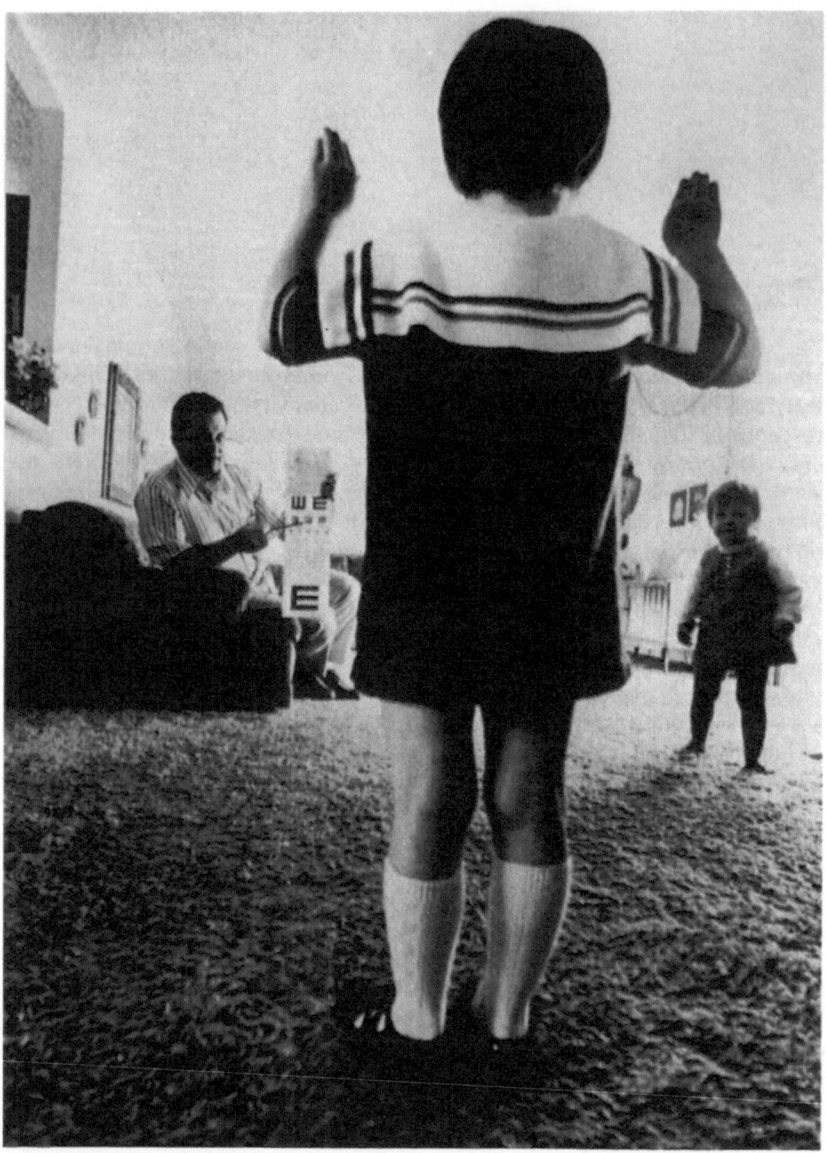

Fig. 1. A father in California is shown giving the Home Eye Test to this five year old daughther as his two year old looks on.

failure only indicates that a child may have a visual defect

We cannot expect to locate through the Home Eye Test, every child who needs eye care.

What we hope for is the chance to locate those thousands of children who have never had their vision tested, who show no outward, obvious sign of eye or vision abnormality, but will demonstrate quite readily in a screening, for example, that they are using only one eye effectively.

The Society's objectives in this program are threefold. First, to identify preschool age children with previously undiagnosed eye conditions. Second, to educate parents to the need for early detection and treatment of vision problems thereby motivating them to seek professional eye care for their child. And third, to inform and gain the involvement of those health professionals who deal with children — general and specialty doctors, nurses, educators and public health officials. Health-care professionals learned about the availability of the test through scientific publications. Actual copies of the test were sent to all ophthalmologists, pediatricians and optometrists, generating a big demand. The Australian College of Ophthalmology's POB Committee has endorsed the test and the Australian Foundation for Prevention of Blindness is printing their own supply. We have utilized a variety of creative devices to promote the Test. We have 20,000 of these counter displays in banks, libraries, health clinics and drug stores. Each display contains post cards for ordering the test and can be sent at no cost to our office. This exhibit has been used at major national conventions such as the American Academy of Ophthalmology and Otolaryngology, and the American Public Health Association.

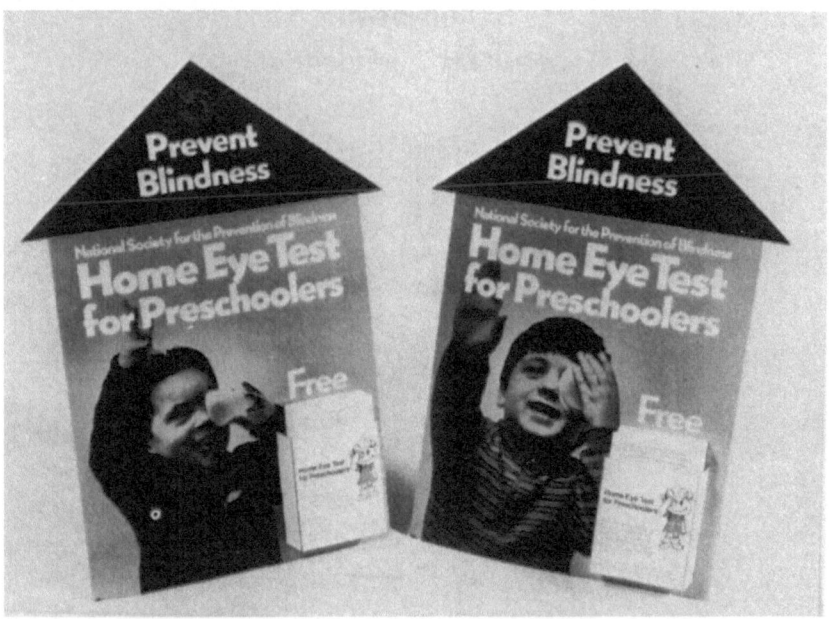

Fig. 2. Thousands of these counter-displays have been placed in banks, drugstores, libraries, health centers and doctor's offices. Individuals can take a postage-free card from the display and order the Home Eye Test.

The Society's community programs reached less than 400,000 children, ages 3-6, during the 1971-1972 screening year. This is less than 3% of the total population in this age group in the U.S. Nearly 18,000 or 5% of these children failed the screening test and were referred for a complete professional eye examination.

As far as the Home Eye Test is concerned, 13,392 results cards have been received. These reports indicated that 5.6% of the children failed the test, that is, could not read the critical line on the chart with one or both eyes. In most instances either the parent had made an appointment for the child to be examined or the child had already been examined. If not, we sent a letter with a pamphlet explaining the need for an examination for all who fail the test.

What type of abnormalities are we finding? The greatest proportion of the children with eye problems (68%) have some type of refractive error.

Amblyopia was found in 15% of the children. This may be reported with a refractive error or strabismus. Muscle imbalance accounted for 14% of the conditions. The remaining 3% are pathologic conditions such as cataract, optic nerve atrophy and degeneration of the retina.

We believe the test has far-reaching significance for it provides a practical method for overcoming shortages of trained personnel, facilities and programs in the search for children with hidden vision problems.

FINDINGS

COMMUNITY PROGRAMS

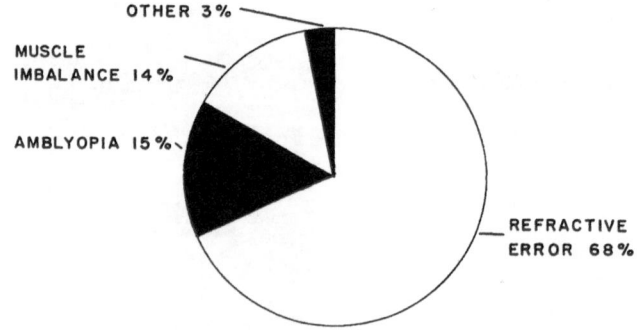

THE EYES IN MULTIPHASIC
HEALTH TESTING

RALPH W. RYAN

(Morgantown, West Virginia, U.S.A.)

Multiphasic health testing is one of the more recently developed medical techniques, which will undoubtedly become more popular and commonplace each year. It has all the advantages of triage or the screening of the public for manifest or incipient disease. Its greatest advantage is in early detection of disease with consequently enhanced opportunities for successful treatment. However, other important advantages are: 1. more efficient utilization of medical manpower and resources because of the decreased load of 'routine' examinations made possible by the screening out of the 'worried wel', 2. decreased cost of medical care from having medical histories and laboratory work done on an 'assembly line' basis by medical assistants and adaptable to computerization if desirable, 3. the possibility of complete case-finding in an entire population, by use of paramedical personnel and 4. conservation of physician time because necessary x-rays, E.C.G.'s and clinical laboratory findings are available on the first visit to the physician so that he can usually make an early diagnosis and begin treatment.

Ophthalmology was probably the first specialty to make widespread use of screening procedures for detection of disease or abnormalities. For years such organizations as the National Society for the Prevention of Blindness and Lions International, together with many local organizations have promoted eye screening of various types, chiefly among school children and older ages of adults. The main object usually was to detect cases of poor visual acuity among the children and insidious and devastating diseases such as glaucoma among older aldults.

I have devoted considerable efforts to develop a battery of screening tests that will yield information to refer patients for medical examination. The equipment requires only medical technicians or even quickly trained clerical employees to operate it. Such testing can be carried out in the ophthalmologist's office, in a mobile unit traveling te remote communities, or incorporated in a laboratory for multiphasic health testing.

The information consists primarily of:

1. Visual 'skills', or characteristics, such as visual acuity at near and distance, the phorias, color vision, etc.
2. The field of vision
3. A test for glaucoma
4. Under some circumstances, it may be desirable to screen for refractive error.

181

The instruments should be as compact and simple to operate as is practical and consistent with accuracy and dependability. Cost is also a consideration. There are a number of instruments available in each of these categories.

Instruments are available for each of the four categories above:

1. A Titmus 'Sight Screener' fitted with selected slides as shown on the attached recording form. Two additional tests not presently provided by Titmus Optical Company can be easily added. These are a 'pinhole' test for the possible improvement of vision by refraction, and a test of fusion using a red-green lens combination with 4 cubes, simulating the Worth 4-dot test.

2. A Harrington-Flocks visual field screener. The reporting form is on the second page of the form for the sight screener.

3. An American Optical Company 'non-contact' tonometer. Recording of the intraocular tension is also on the second page of the Titmus recording form.

4. A 'Diotron', as representative of the refractive screening devices. The recording of refractive error screening is on the second page of the form for the sight screener.

The Titmus Sight Screener recording form provides for recording results by circling the scores by approriately coded colors in pencil or ink. Thus the findings made without glasses are to be recorded by making a circle with black ink around the appropriate scores. Red ink is similarly used to circle the scores while lenses (either spectacle or contact) are worn. Green is used for distance vision scores while a +1.75 blurring lens is inserted in the screener to detect persons with a high degree of hyperopia or 'farsightedness'. This helps find the cases which may have good visual acuity but are subject to eye fatigue because of a need to accomodate for distance. This could conceivably be used in near vision to show that there is a presbyopia correctable by plus lenses. Blue ink is used to circle the scores while a 'pinhole lens' is inserted in the screener; if visual acuity is improved by looking through the 'pinhole' opening, then improvement of vision by glasses can be expected; if there is no improvement in a case with poor visual acuity, then organic basis for the poor vision can be suspected. The pinhole lenses are not presently routinely furnished by Titmus but may be placed in the holder designed for the +1.75 lenses. Red, yellow and blue colors are to be recognized on the first far-vision slide.

The slides number 1 and 9 for distance (far) visual acuity may thus have recordings in all 4 code colors of black without lenses, red with lenses, green with added +1.75 blurring lenses, and blue with pinhole lenses. The near vision slides number 7 and 11 might be scored in black, red and blue and even green.

Number 2 slide records in prism diopters the vertical phorias or tendency of one eye to deviate above the other at distance. Cases may occur in which uncorrected eyes show a vertical phoria which is circled in black. If the patient's glasses contain a prism correction, then red ink may be used to show the score with the corrective prism in the glasses.

Slide 3 records any tendency for the eye to deviate horizontally, either nasally or temporally. Again, recording may be made with or without glasses

182

by using black or red ink. In addition the +1.75 lens may produce change in the horizontal phorias which may be of interest in certain cases. These would be recorded in green.

Slide 4 shows whether fusion is normal by visualizing 3 cubes. Simultaneously fixation is indicated if 4 cubes are seen, and suppression of one eye if only 2 cubes are seen. When a red lens is inserted over one eye in the tester and a green lens over the other, the cube ordinarily seen as white assumes the color of the lens which is in front of the dominant eye. (The red-green lens combination can be furnished by special order, in a holder made for the +1.75 lenses).

Slide 5 shows patterns seen as having varying degrees of elevation if stereopsis is present. Correction of the eye with glasses may produce a better score if there is significant refractive error. Appropriate colors must be used in circling scores.

Slide 6 contains color patterns typical of the Ishihara plates. Corrected vision by lenses or pinhole may give a better score if a significant refractive error is present.

Slide 7 involves near vision. The scores of persons with high hyperopia or presbyopia may be poor unless glasses are worn.

Slide 8 involves the tendency to deviate horizontally in near vision.

The slides for small children and illiterates begin with 9 which contains various sized pictures which should be recognized by the 4 year old. Letters are also present to find if the child can recognize them. Again the various colors must be used in circling the scores for uncorrected vision, corrected vision, the +1.75 lens for excessive hyperopia (far-sightedness), and the pinhole lens to show that uncorrected poor vision can be improved with glasses.

Slide 10 shows whether there is a tendency for deviation of the eyes, either horizontally or vertically. If the apple is falling on the table, the tendency to deviation is within limits considered normal. Left or right positions of the apple would denote esophoria or exophoria respectively, the left or right eye having a tendency to deviate upward in fixation.

Slide 11 is an E. chart with the child required to show which way the legs of the E. point, down, up, right or left. The slide also has colored letters for recognition of both the color and the letter. Again scoring must be with appropriate colors of ink.

Slide 12 is similar to 10 but with values of deviation appropriate for near vision.

The visual field device has pages with spots of paint which glow under ultraviolet light. The patient places his chin on the chin-rest and one eye is occluded. He fixates on a target in center of the page with the uncovered eye. An ultra-violet light is flashed on for an instant and he must say how many spots he saw. As the pages are turned and the test continued, spots are shown in areas covering the entire chart. Gross field defects are detected by this instrument and later should be delineated more minutely by the common visual field devices. If the patient does not demonstrate a defect in the field at the point coinciding with his optic nerve, the physiological blind spot, the field recording is less significant.

The American Optical non-contact tonometer has the advantage that it

Circle the scores with:
Black ink if checked without lenses
Red ink if checked with lenses
Green ink if +1.75 lenses are inserted
Blue ink if pinhole lenses are inserted

Name_____

Date_____Examiner_____

ADULT VISION FINDINGS

Slides (1) SL-AF-2 Far Vision	Right	20/200	R	Left	20/200	S
		20/100	VN		20/100	CK
		20/70	KCSZ		20/70	RVCN
	Yellow	20/50	SVORN		20/50	DKNOV
	Red	20/40	VSKCDH		20/40	RCZHDS
	Blue	20/30	DKVSNOR		20/30	SROKVCN
		20/25	ZVCDSRH		20/25	HDZVROK
		20/20	SCHKVROZ		20/20	ZKCSVONR
		20/15	KDZCVSOHR		20/15	SOZNDKCVH

(2) VPF-1 Far	Vert. Phorias in Pr. Diop.	1 1½ LH	2 1 LH	3 ½ LH	4 0	5 ½ RH	6 1 RH	7 1½ RH

(3) LPF-1 Far	Lat. Phor. in Pr. Diop.	1 7es	2 6es	3 5es	4 4es	5 3es	6 2es	7 1es	8 0	9 1ex	10 2ex	11 3ex	12 4ex	13 5ex	14 6ex	15 7ex

(4) F-F-1 Far	Red and Green lenses: White cube takes color of lens over the dominant eye. Dominance: Right Left Neither (Circle One)
	Fusion 3 Cubes 4 Cubes 2 Cubes
	Normal Simultan. Fix. Suppression 1 eye

(5) SDF-1 Stereop. Tests Far	Elevated Pattern	1 B	2 L	3 B	4 T	5 T	6 L	7 R	8 L	9 R
	% Fusion Shepherd-Fry	15%	30%	50%	60%	70%	80%	85%	90%	95%
	Angle of Ster. in seconds of Arc.	400	200	100	70	50	40	30	25	20

(6) CDF-1 Color Vision Far	Ishihari	12	5, 26	6 16
	Isochromatic Plates	Color Deficient	Impaired Red-Green	Indust. Stand.

(7) SL-AN-1 Near	Right	14/140	J-14	N	Left	J-14	H
		14/70	J-14	RS		J-14	ZD
		14/49	J-11	VDKO		J-11	CHRS
		14/35	J-6	RNHKS		J-6	VCDNZ
		14/28	J-3	SCVZOD		J-3	NOVKCH
		14/21	J-2	ZSHRKCV		J-2	KDRVONS
		14/17.5	J-2	KOCNRSD		J-2	SZRCHKN
		14/14	J-1	DROKSNVH		J-1	HVOSRZDC
		14/10.5	J-1	VRNCKOHDZ		J-1	RKVZDNHCS

(8) LPN-1 Lateral Phor. in Pr. Diop. Near	1	2	3	4	5	6	7	8	9	10	11	12	13	14	15
	10½ es	4 es	7½ es	6 es	4½ es	3 es	1½ es	0	1½ ex	3 ex	4½ ex	6 ex	7½ ex	9 ex	10½ ex

184

Name_____

Date_____ Examiner_____

Circle the scores with:
Black ink if checked without lenses
Red ink if checked with lenses
Green ink if +1.75 lenses are inserted
Blue ink if pinhole lenses are inserted

Children Vision Findings

Slides (9) AF-APS-1 Picture Chart Far	Right Top		(Auto, Telephone, Cake, Horse)	Left Top		(Auto, Telephone, Cake, Horse)
		20/100	A. T. C. H.		20/100	A. T. C. H.
Picture	A	20/50	H. C. T. A.	A	20/50	C. H. A. T.
Chart	B	20/40	C. A. H. T.	B	20/40	T. C. H. A.
Far	C	20/30	T. H. A. C.	C	20/30	H. A. T. C.

(10) PF-S-1 Phorias Far	Apple on Table		Apple off Table	
				Above
			Left	Right
		Normal		Below

(11) AN-BRL-1 E			Right		Left		
	Blue A	14/35	J-6	DUR UDR	14/35	J-6	UDR DUR
Chart Near Vision	Red B	14/28	J-3	UDR LRU	14/28	J-3	LDR UDR
	Yellow C	14/21	J-2	RUL DUD	12/21	J-2	DLU RUL
	Green D	14/14	J-1	DLU RLU	14/14	J-1	RUL DLU

(12) PN-S-1 Phorias Near	Apple on Table		Apple off Table	
				Above
			Left	Right
		Normal		Below

HARRINGTON-FLOCKS SCREENING FIELDS

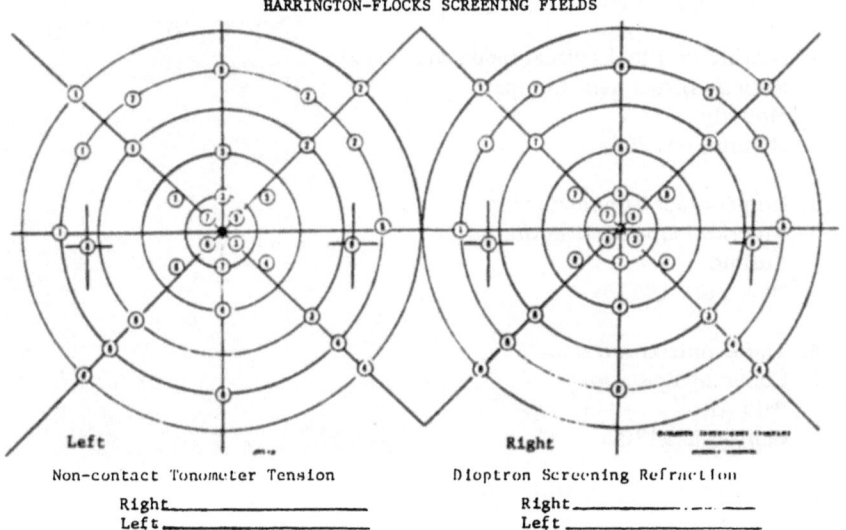

Left   Right

Non-contact Tonometer Tension   Dioptron Screening Refraction

Right_____   Right_____
Left _____   Left _____

touches the eye only with a small jet of clean air, thus making it a good instrument for technician use. Optical devices record the minute indentation of the cornea by the jet of air, giving a reading in terms of milimeters of mercury on a dial. Readings are claimed by the manufacturer to approximate those of the Schiotz tonometer. They are recorded on the second page of the Titmus form.

The instrument is first tried on the closed eyelids or hand of the patient to get him accustomed to the snap and feel of the jet of air being discharged. We have found most patients still hold their eyelids tense and exert some pressure on the eye. This can be relieved by asking the patient to stare at the tiny target light with both eyes as wide open as possible and the forehead wrinkled. The forehead must be held tightly against the head rest to permit the instrument to function. Mascara on eyelashes sometimes clogs the tiny orifice from which the air jet emerges, thus blocking the action of the instrument.

The Dioptron makes screening measurements of both the spherical and astigmatic refractive error of the eyes. It is capable of being operated by a technician. If no cycloplegia is used, the patient should be urged to fixate in such way as to simulate distance fixation as much as possible. Ordinarily no attempt is made to measure the refractive error involved in near or reading vision by such a screening instrument.

Instruments used may be procured from the following sources in the United States:

1. Titmus sight screener
   Titmus Optical Company
   P.O. Box 191
   Petersburg, Virginia 23803

2. Harrington-Flocks visual field screener
   Roberts Instrument Company
   Moberly
   Missouri 65270

3. Non-contact Tonometer
   American Optical Corporation
   Buffalo
   New York 14214

4. The Dioptron refractor
   Coherent Radiations
   Palo Alto
   California 94302.

MASS SCREENING OF OCULAR TENSION BASED ON COMPUTER ANALYSIS OF NORMAL EYES

YOSHIHIKO SHIOSE,

(Nagoya, Japan)

In glaucoma screening, twenty millimeters of mercury has been generally accepted, as the upper limit of normal ocular tension.

The validity of this criterion has been statistically established. This criterion, however, is not universally valid as the measure for ocular tension, because numerous additional factors must also be considered.

The present study was undertaken to confirm the normal value of ocular tension under diverse conditions. Age, sex and the laterality of the eyes were taken into consideration in an attempt to obtain correlations between ocular tension and systemic factors. Attempts were also made to find acceptable methods that may serve for the estimation of the normal intraocular pressure.

SUBJECTS AND METHODS

Normal ocular tensions were measured on 29,896 eyes of 14,968 subjects examined. They formed part of our Automated Multiphasic Health Testing (AMHT) system during the year 1972. The subjects selected were healthy individuals who had no medical complaints, and no physical abnormalities.

Measurements of ocular tension using standardization Schioetz tonometers were carried out twice on both left and right eyes. The tests were performed by eight experienced examiners.

The data obtained was analyzed on an IBM 360/Model 40 computer.

RESULTS AND COMMENTS

I. Normal values of ocular tension

Statistics on 29,896 eyes revealed that the normal value of ocular tension was 15.3 corresponding to 2.40 mm. Hg.

Detailed results of the relationship between ocular tensions, sex and age appear on Table 1. This table illustrates three outstanding factors that influenced mean values; 1). Ocular tension of females was higher than that of males regardless of age or the eye tested; 2). the ocular tension of the left eye was higher than that of the right eye regardless of age or sex; 3). the ocular tension tended to be lower with increasing age regardless of sex of the right or left eye.

TABLE I

MEAN AND VARIATION OF OCULAR TENSION IN NORMAL HUMAN EYES

MALE:

Age Group		-20	20-	30-	40-	50-	60-	70-	Total
Number		16	517	2778	4752	2497	953	157	11678
R.E	M	16.3	14.9	15.0	14.9	14.6	14.5	14.2	14.8
	S.D.	2.08	2.62	2.48	2.52	2.69	2.79	3.03	2.59
L.E	M	16.9	15.6	15.7	15.6	15.3	15.2	14.7	15.5
	S.D.	2.41	2.58	2.46	2.59	2.70	3.13	2.88	2.64

FEMALE:

Age Group		-20	20-	30-	40-	50-	60-	70-	Total
Number		20	234	632	1164	884	305	31	3270
R.E	M	15.7	15.5	15.3	15.3	15.3	14.9	14.3	15.3
	S.D.	1.66	2.31	2.30	2.32	2.55	2.50	2.70	2.40
L.E	M	15.8	16.1	16.0	16.1	16.0	15.6	14.7	16.0
	S.D.	1.92	2.33	2.24	2.23	2.60	2.84	3.44	2.42

RELATIONSHIP BETWEEN I.O.P. AND AGE

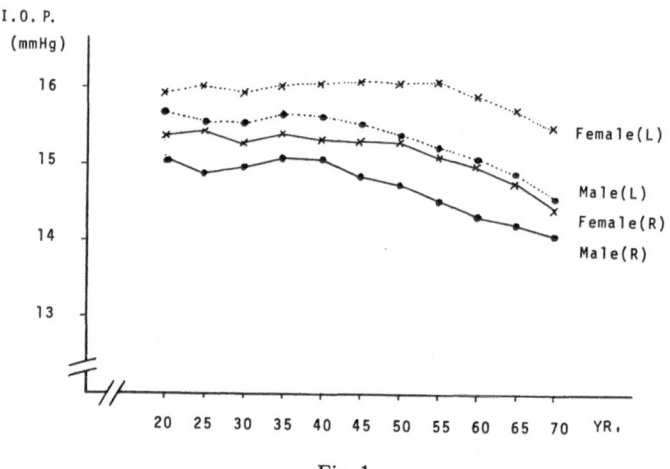

Fig. 1.

These results are shown on Figure 1.

The highest mean occular tension was noted in female-left eyes. This was followed by male-left eyes, female-right eyes, and male-right eyes.

' Figure 2 shows frequency distribution curves in respect to sex and the two eyes. Standard deviations (SD) of both eyes were close in value in both males and females. The curves obtained from left eyes were 0.7 mm. Hg. higher than those from right eyes. In comparing ocular tensions of the two

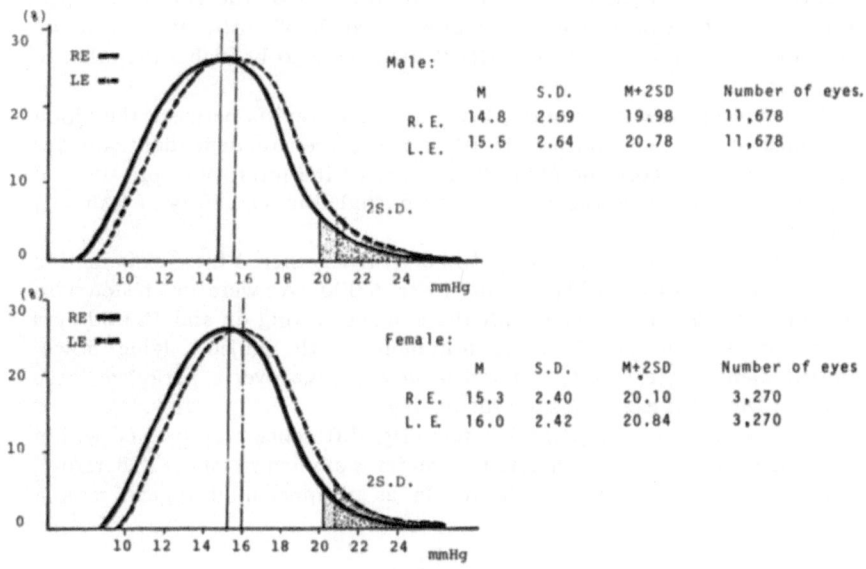

Fig. 2.

TABLE II
Upper Limits of the normal Tension (2SD)
Total: 29,896 eyes

Male:

Age	20–	30-	40-	50-	60-	70-
RE	20.14	19.96	19.94	19.98	20.08	20.00
LE	20.76	20.62	20.78	20.70	21.46	20.46

Female

Age	20-	30-	40-	50-	60-	70-
RE	20.12	19.90	19.94	20 40	19.90	19.70
LE	20.76	20.46	20.56	21.20	21.28	21.58

sexes, there was 0.5 mm. Hg. difference in the mean values in both right and left eyes.

Application of t-tests yielded a highly significant difference ($p < 0.01$) in ocular tensions between right and left eyes of males (−20.5), females (−11.7), male and female right eyes (−23.8), and male and female left eyes (−9.7).

The results were characteristic and regular as far as the mean values were concerned. The upper limit of normal tension modified with 2SD rose to 20 mm. Hg. regardless of age and sex (Table II and Figure 2).

189

In comparison, the laterality of ocular tensions between the right and left eyes appeared rather distinct. This may be explained on the basis of anatomical asymmetry that exists at the bifurcation of the carotid arteries. Since the left carotid artery is a direct branch of aortic arc, the blood pressure of the left ophthalmic artery is expected to be higher than that of the right.

If we accept the assumption that a difference exists between the blood pressures of the two ophthalmic arteries, the pressure-dependent aqueous inflow will show corresponding differences in the intraocular pressures of the two sides. These considerations must exclude the possibility of technical bias.

Consistent results were obtained in statistics gathered from examination of 18,000 eyes during 1971. During 1971, 6,000 eyes were also tested with the Mackey-Mark tonometer with the subjects sitting up and 12,000 eyes were tested with the Schioetz tonometer with subjects lying down. Measurements were carried out twice on each eye over a period of three months. Different examiners did the testing.

From a clinical standpoint 1-2 mm. Hg. difference may be well within range of error when the Schioetz tonometer is applied to an eye. Therefore, the conventional standard of 20 mm.Hg. as an upper limit appears reasonable.

II. Correlation between ocular tensions and systemic factors

Attempts were made on all subjects to obtain primary regression coefficients between the left ocular tension and 42 items chosen from the Automated Multiphasic Health Testing system.

Figure 3 demonstrates 19 items which have high correlations to the left ocular tension. Yet, the coefficient of the right tension to that of the left is extraordinarily high, amounting to +0.78779. Ponderal index, the degree of obesity, diastolic and systolic blood pressure occupy even higher ranks. Age was found to have a negative correlation to the left ocular tension at the rank 8. Here, the ponderal index is calculated by height/$^3\sqrt{\text{weight}}$. The degree of obesity is expressed by the percentage ratio of virtual weight to the standard weight obtained by 0.9 (height - 100).

A correlation histogram of the left ocular tension and several items of higher rank was prepared.

Figure 4 shows the frequency distribution curves of systolic blood pressures in relation to varied levels of left ocular tension.

Figure 4 reveals that a steady correlation between ocular tension and blood pressure exists. As the ocular tension increased to 10, 12, 14, and 20 mm. Hg., respectively, corresponding increases of the blood pressure took place. When the ocular tension exceeded 20 mm. Hg. the distribution curves tended to be pushed back towards lower values. The systolic and diastolic blood pressure as well as the degree of obesity displayed similar patterns. These facts suggest that within the normal range, ocular tension increases proportionally to the blood pressure and the degree of obesity. This rule, however, does not apply when the ocular tension exceeds 20 mm. Hg.

According to our observations, advanced glaucoma is frequently ac-

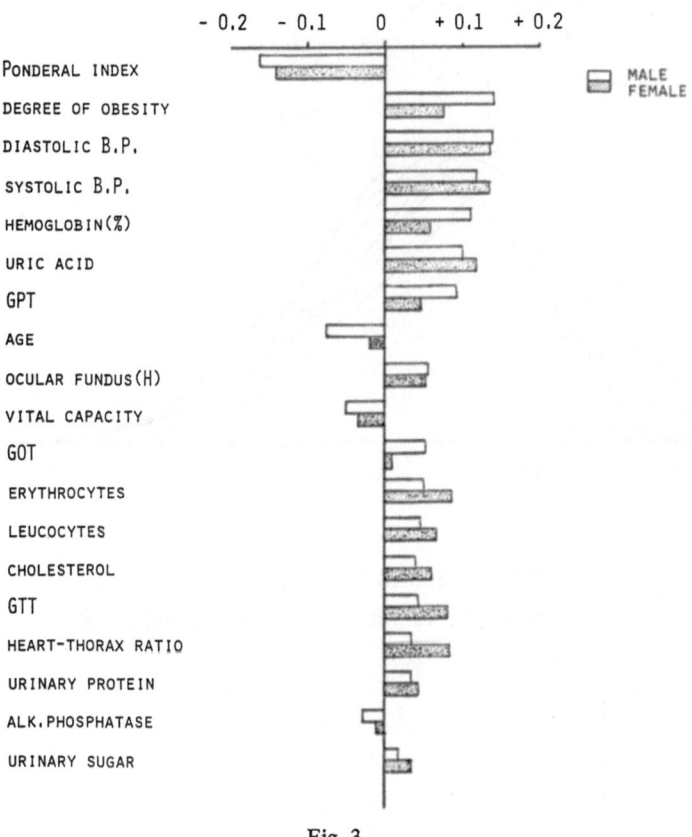

RANKING OF PRIMARY REGRESSION COEFFICIENTS OF SYSTEMIC FACTORS
IN RESPECT TO THE I.O.P.

Fig. 3.

companied by systemic hypotension and a slender stature.

Another type of analysis was attempted by producing a percentage scatter diagram of the left ocular tension and systolic blood pressure based on a correlation histogram (Fig. 5). According to this, four phases may be postulated utilizing the upper limit of normal ocular tension and the lower limit of blood pressure (97.5th percentile—: 1). The 'normal tension phase' expresses an equilibrium between blood pressure and ocular tension. 2). 'Relative low tension phase' is characterized by normal ocular tension with relatively low blood pressure 3). 'Proportionate high tension phase' has high ocular tension over 20 mm. Hg. with proportionally high blood pressure. 4). 'Relative high tension phase' is characterized by high ocular tension with relatively low blood pressure. Similar throughts could be applied to other factors which hold high correlations with ocular tension. The validity of such assumptions must await further investigations.

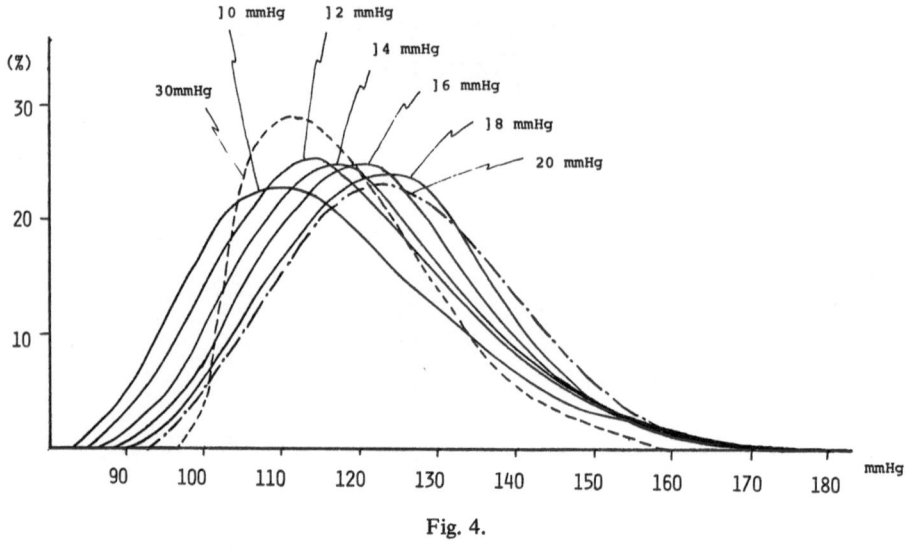

PERCENTAGE DISTRIBUTION OF L-I.O.P. CURVES
RELATIVE TO THE SYSTOLIC BLOOD PRESSURE

Fig. 4.

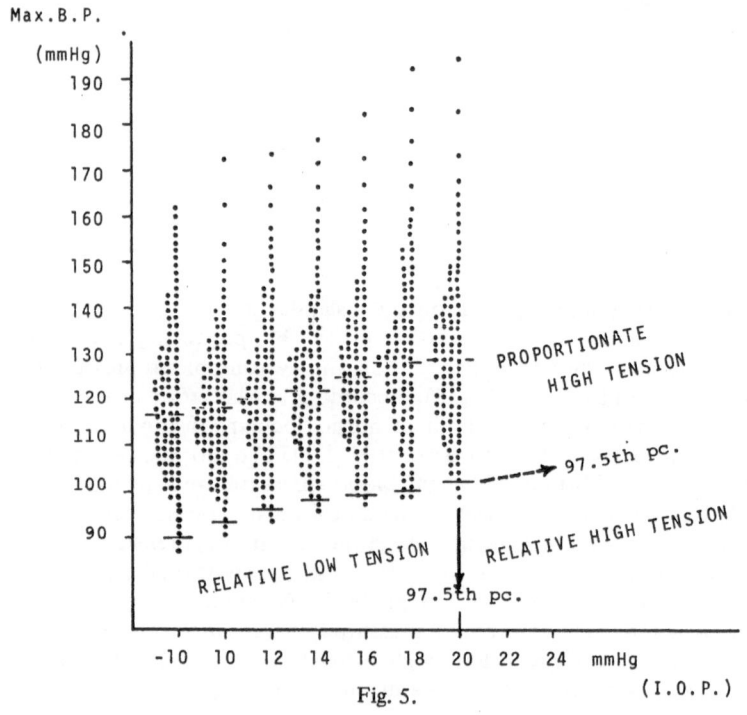

PERCENTAGE SCATTER DIAGRAMM OF L-I.O.P.
RELATIVE TO THE SYSTOLIC BLOOD PRESSURE

Fig. 5.

III. 'Ocular-Blood pressure index' (IOP/BP ratio)

Using ocular tension as the sole index for glaucoma screening, it appears reasonable to employ 20 mm. Hg. as the upper limit. This is despite the fact that the distribution of ocular tension is different when different factors are involved.

Attempts were undertaken to plot the percentage ratio of ocular tension, and diastolic blood pressure against age (Fig. 6).

As shown in Fig. 6, 'the index' had a trend to decrease with increasing age. 'The index' of females was higher than that of males in all age groups. These phenomena may be explained on the basis of the diastolic blood pressure increasing with age whereas the ocular tension is decreasing. The ocular pressure is higher in females than in males. Blood pressure is higher in males than in females.

PERCENTAGE REPRESENTATION OF L-I.O.P./
DIASTOLIC BLOOD PRESSURE RATIO FOR AGE

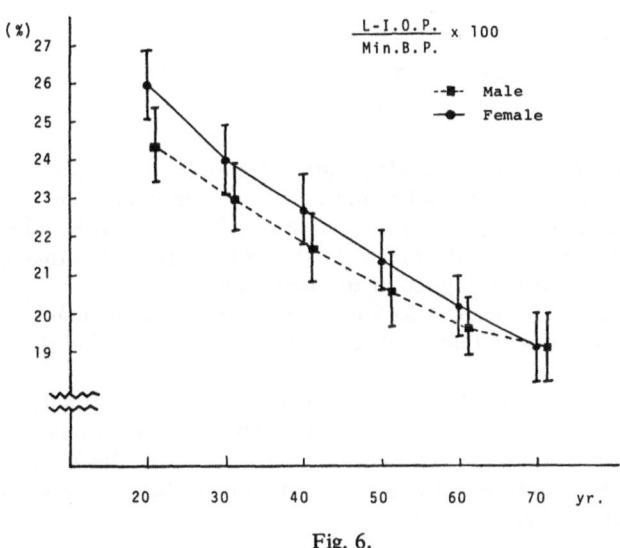

Fig. 6.

Using the mean value of 'the index', it is possible to compute the mean ocular tension of a subject whose diastolic pressure is known. Assuming the diastolic blood pressure to be 70 mm. Hg. the mean ocular tension of 20th female would be 18.2 mm. Hg. and that of 70th would be 13.3 mm. Hg. respectively.

Aqueous is largely dependent on ocular hemodynamics in terms of production and outflow systems. Blood circulation of the optic nervehead and the peripapillary choroid are influenced by ocular tension. It appears that under normal conditions there exists a steady state between the ocular tension and the blood pressure.

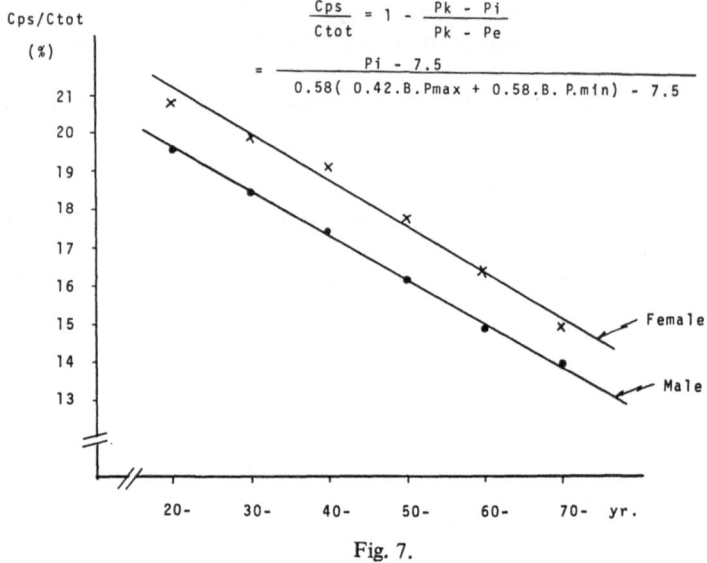

Fig. 7.

Figure 7 illustrates the percentage ratio of pseudofacility (Cps) to total facility (Ctot) estimated by Goldmann's equation. The results obtained were in accord with those measured by the pressure cuff method of Kupfer.

The similarity between 'the index' and Cps/Ctot ratio shows that aging is the most conspicuous limiting factor to these values.

Since all biological phenomena are more or less age-dependent, it is not unreasonable to suggest that the age factor should be included into the evaluation of glaucomas.

The validity of 'the index' should be checked in known normal groups as well as in patients with ocular hypertension. These investigations are still in progress. Although a number of factors must be studied, the acceptance of 'the index' would supply additional information to the currently available standards of ocular hypertension.

ACKNOWLEDGEMENT

The author wishes to thank DR. TOHRU IWATSUKA for providing valuable data, and to DR. NOBORU OKAMOTO for help with computer programming.

OPTICAL TELE-CAMERA

J.F. CUENDET

(Lausanne, Switzerland)

PRINCIPLES OF APPARATUS

The Optical Tele-Camera is a closed-circuit television system allowing the enlargement of a document up to 50 times. Therefore, this enlargement is far greater than the one obtained by traditional optical means. This system enables some partially sighted patients to read and write.

Besides the great enlargement, this modality conveys the image of a document in the negative. The contrast is indeed better when the message appears white on a dark background. The patient must concentrate on the text and not on the surroundings.

However, pictures have to be seen in the positive; therefore, by means of a simple switch, it is possible to change instantaneously from one to the other. Another switch allows distance reading on a screen or a black board. A special accessory allows the patient to view what is being typed. Finally, several TV screens can be connected to the same camera. This has proved to be very useful for teaching classes of partially sighted children.

DIFFERENT MODELS OBTAINABLE ON THE MARKET

As a result of the pioneer work of SAMUEL M. GENENSKI, the first apparatus was put on the market in January, 1971, in California. It was called VISUALTEK. Since then other apparatuses were designed. They include the MAKROLECTOR 140 made in Switzerland and the REINECKER made in Germany. The latter two present advantages of less dazzling, fixation of a document with magnetic devices, and good maintenance service. Prices vary between US $1,500,00 and $3,000.00. Our personal experience is based only on the VISUALTEK.

VISUAL REQUIREMENTS

The minimal required visual acuity is 1/60, 20/1200, or counting fingers at 1 meter. If the visual field is constricted, a small screen, 10" x 7", may be used. In most cases a domestic TV screen can be used.

TECHNICAL REQUIREMENTS

The subject must show sufficient technical ability to handle the various buttons that regulate brilliancy, contrast, diaphragm, sharpness, zoom and

195

illumination angle of the document.

Persons over 70 years of age find it difficult to operate these technical devices. Therefore, they can scarcely benefit from them. If old people require assistance to adjust the buttons, it would be more practical for them to hire an assistant as a reader.

PSYCHOLOGICAL REQUIREMENTS

The great enlargement of the text shows up only single words, part of a word, or even isolated letters at a time. Therefore, special psychological adaptive abilities are necessary to coordinate successive parts of the text to make a comprehensible sentence. A given reading speed is advisable. Intellectual persons do better than those who have only minimal education.

CONCLUSIONS

The Optical Tele-Camera is of great value to certain partially sighted individuals whose visual acuity ranges from 20/100 to 20/1200. They must not be too old and should show some minimal technical abilities and be able to make psychological adjustments. The high cost of the apparatus keeps most of the potential beneficiaries from purchasing it. Therefore, it is recommended that the organizations for social welfare buy them for persons or groups of persons whose vision cannot be helped by other means.

I propose that the International Association for Prevention of Blindness should make definite recommendations on behalf of organizations for social welfare in order that the latter may assume financing of Optical Tele-Cameras all over the world, so we will reach one of our social goals: to enable persons with severe visual impairments to read.

EDUCATIONAL IMPLICATIONS OF
MANPOWER PLANNING IN
PUBLIC HEALTH OPHTHALMOLOGY

B. NIZETIC

(Copenhagen, Denmark)

Prevention of blindness is a confusing term that means different things to different people.

The concept of public health ophthalmology imposes a radical, prospective change in the traditional role of the clinical ophthalmologist. In addition to his expert clinical performance and the creation of new models of ocular molecular biology, he has to participate in the search for new models of eye-health care delivery, in close cooperation with allied eye-health personnel and other relevant disciplines. He has to do this within the context of the existing public health system in the country where he practices.

This change in the traditional role is necessary, because the gap is widening between the best which ophthalmology could offer and that which is actually available to populations at large.

The public health approach to problems of visual impairment and blindness implies the acceptance and implementation of the following concepts:
1. Public health ophthalmology implies a change from crisis or acute intervention to comprehensive eye-health care. The latter includes, in a continuum, prevention, cure and rehabilitation of the visually impaired.
2. Public health ophthalmology is problem-oriented. This means that the ultimate goal of reducing or eliminating disability due to visual impairment and blindness ought to be broken down into a number of objectives concerning comprehensive eye-health care. These onjectives must be met by different programs and projects. The advantage of programmed projects lies in the fact that they require a preliminary, explicit statement concerning the following parameters:
   a. objectives of the program or project
   b. methodology to be applied
   c. population covered by the program
   d. time allocated to the program
   e. manpower necessary to run the program or project with detailed role descriptions and supervision patterns
   f. methodology for the evaluation of the program — efficiency and effectiveness.

Consideration of these points is expected to lead to greatly improved programs and more rational decision making.
3. The team concept is basic to public health ophthalmology. It implies the

coordinated utilization of different skills within the speciality as well as the utilization of skills from multidisciplinary specialties.

4. Public health ophthalmology includes epidemiology, modern management procedures, and clinical knowledge. This concept is both a science and a service. Its service dimension, as well as the critical team approach, makes the concept of planning and its associated field of evaluation mandatory.

The justification for planning and evaluation is based on the assumption that all current health actions have repercusssions on the future health status of a population. In addition, these measures have cumulative effects on social expectations and demands for services. Furthermore, it must be remembered that the creation of new resources, such as skilled manpower, requires time. The most effective and efficient use of resources is also necessary because of the steady increase in costs in the health sector. Planning is not the speciality of a few experts, but a 'must' for all decision-makers. Ophthalmologists, too, are called upon to act as decision-makers for services regarding their responsibilities or to act as technical advisers in general health planning teams. Their role is essential in guaranteeing the application of high standards and in protecting the interests of eye-health professionals and their clients.

The foregoing considerations have the following educational implications:

1. What are the objectives of teaching public health ophthalmology?

The educational problem in public health ophthalmology consists of training a sufficient number of eye-health professionals at different levels, who will be able to conduct comprehensive eye-health services in the most economical way. In addition, there is a need to spread ophthalmological knowledge to other professions which are involved in eye-health care.

2. What should courses in public health ophthalmology encompass?

In addition to clinical aspects, matters pertaining to ophthalmoepidemiology and eye-health practice research should be included.

a. Clinical aspects of eye-health: Diagnostic and treatment procedures and relevant teaching in the basic sciences already from the core of the usual curriculum in clinical ophthalmology.

b. Ophthalmo-epidemiology: Two underlying facts support the teaching of ophthalmo-epidemiology to medical students.

First, the changing patterns of eye diseases and the increasing importance of organizing scarce resources have made it necessary for the medical student to have an elementary knowledge of eye-health epidemiological patterns and statistics and to know enough about public health ophthalmology to be able to evaluate and plan.

Secondly, the teaching of epidemiology could help ensure the needed emphasis on diseases that are common in the community as opposed to those seen principally in hospitals.

198

c. Eye-health practice research: Eye-health practice[1] research is concerned with organizational problems: planning, management, logistics and the delivery of eye-health care services.

The following list of priority areas illustrates the problems that are encountered in eye-health practice research:

1. Manpower: Personnel utilization, in studying the best balance between ophthalmologists, nurses and other eye-health personnel in different types of services;

Systematic studies of the education and training needed by different categories of personnel in the eye-health-care team when their respective functions and activities are rationalized and, in particular, the education required for the team leader, an ophthalmologist.

2. Organization: Comparison of the relative advantages of separating medical care of ophthalmic patients and personal preventive eye care and of providing integrated, personal eye-health care.

3. Utilization: Ophthalmic bed utilization and other utilization studies.

4. Major Problem Areas: Studies to identify the best lines of attack on major communicable eye diseases, nutritional blindness, glaucoma, ocular trauma, and others considered to be of local or regional importance.

5. Quality of eye-health care: Evaluation of the quality of eye-health care.

6. Cost: Cost-effectiveness and cost-benefit studies, e.g., studies of the cost of certain categories of eye disease to the community and of the cost of eye disease control systems.

7. Terminology, information and research systems, indices, statistical methods in ophthalmology:

a). The standardization of terminology for eye-health care items, categories of personnel, eye-health care institutions, etc.

b). The development of indicators of levels of eye-health and eye-health care provision.

8. Need/Demand: Eye-health care provision and the need/demand relationship.

How should relevant public health factors in ophthalmology be taught?

Developments in educational theory obligue us to seek solutions in close collaboration with specialists in this field. Clinical excellence is not enough to guarantee appropriate teaching. Classical methods of instruction need to be complemented by newer means. Integrated teaching for various health professions is recommended for public health ophthalmological training. Further analysis and studies are necessary. Closer cooperation between ophthalmologists, health planners, and specialists in medical education is highly recommended.

[1] The practice of public health ophthalmology includes provision of traditional public health ophthalmological services: comunicable eye disease control of environmental eye-health hazards, and the planning, administration and management of all forms of personal eye-health care. Within this field lie personal preventive services, eye-health surveillance, screening, diagnosis, treatment and restorative services in hospitals and in the community.

Undergraduate, postgraduate and continuing education form an indivisible whole.

a. Undergraduate training in ophthalmology: The effective participation of general practitioners and students of allied professions in the delivery of comprehensive eye-health care requires that they become familar with the concepts of public health ophthalmology. Epidemiological patterns of blinding conditions need particular emphasis.

b. Postgraduate curriculum in ophthalmology: The study of ophthalmo-epidemiology and eye-health practice research round out classical clinical knowledge and skills.

Research work in the field invariably needs collaboration of clinical practitioners and other health personnel. Surveys, organizational research methods, and multidisciplinary research projects should be incorporated into postgraduate training of ophthalmologists.

c. Continuing education: There is a close relationship between the curriculum of continuing education and that of basic and postgraduate in ophthalmology. They cannot be developed independent of each other if they are to be relevant to the eye-health problems and needs of each country.

REFERENCES

NINZETIC, B. Sur les aspects 'santé publique' des problèmes de la vision et des maladies, oculaires au Meroc (Essai d'une approche globale devant servir comme base a l'établissement d'un plan d'ensemble dans le domaine de l'ophthalmologic. Unpublished WHO/EURO document, March 1970.

NIZETIC, B. Perspectives in Ophthalmology – A Public Health Point of View. *Canad. J. Ophthal.,* 8: *311* (1973).

NIZETIC, B. Prevention of 'Blindness' – Potentialities of a Systems Analaysis Approach, *Acta Ophthalmologica,* 52: *134* (1974).

Public Health Ophthalmology in the European Region, by Dr. B. NIZETIC, reprinted from Public Health in Europe, No.2, Wld Hlth Org., Regional Office for Europe, Copenhagen, 1973.

The Prevention of Blindness, Report of a WHO Study Group, Wld. Hlth. Or. Techn. Rep. Ser., 1973, No. 518.

PREVENTIVE OPHTHALMOLOGY:
A UNIT WITHIN A MEDICAL SCHOOL

I.C. MICHAELSON

(Jerusalem, Israel)

Preventive medicine, while concerned originally with communicable disease and nutrition has in recent years become concerned also with the aging and degenerative processes including the cardio-vascular diseases. While the primary phase of its development is still the main concern of preventists in developing countries, the latter phase is most practised in the developed countries, its practitioners being essentially trained in internal medicine. They are active in the services supplied by public health bodies; or are engaged essentially in research and teaching in a department of public health or a department of social medicine of a medical school. These departments are separate from, although in many ways parallel to, the department of medicine of the medical school. They have their own programmes, staffs and budgets.

There is, however, a great part of disease, as classified into the specialities, which is somewhat neglected in medical schools so far as organised teaching and research in prevention are concerned. The purpose of this report is to describe the programme and beginning activities of a unit of preventive ophthalmology with the Hebrew University Medical School of Jerusalem. It is hoped, if its pioneer activities and programme are better known, that they may stimulate similar departments for prevention elsewhere in ophthalmology and in other specialities.

JERUSALEM INSTITUTE FOR THE PREVENTION OF BLINDNESS AND OCULAR DISEASE

The Institute is housed in the heart of Jerusalem in the Strauss Health Centre which is a part of the Hadassah Medical Organisation. The basic reason for its establishment is that probably at least half of the blindness in developing countries and about 20% of the blindness in developed countries could have been avoided. There are about 6000 blind persons in Israel. The following is a description of the Institute's programme which is indicated on the accompanying diagram.

The personnel consists of ophthalmologists, epidemiologist, biostatistician and secretaries. In many important ways the staff is counselled by the department of Social Medicine of the Hebrew University Medical School. The Israel Ophthalmological Society is closely identified with the work of the Institute and its members already have 8 years of experience in a national cooperative study in the prevention of retinal detachment.

201

JERUSALEM INSTITUTE FOR PREVENTION OF BLINDNESS

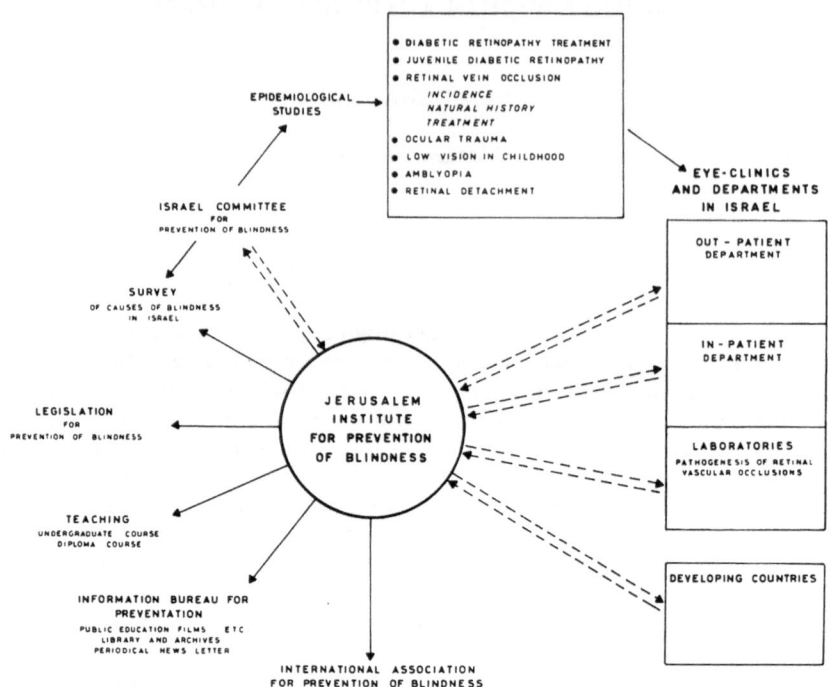

Diagram illustrating the activities of the Jerusalem Institute for the Prevention of Blindness.

COOPERATIVE EPIDEMIOLOGICAL RESEARCHES

The Institute has organised a survey of all cases of blindness in Israel and of low vision in childhood. It is planning seven different national or regional projects whose objects are the investigation of the incidence, natural history, pathogenesis or preventive therapy of such causes of blindness as detachment of the retina, retinal vein occlusion, certain genetic disorders, ocular trauma, diabetic retinopathy and amblyopia. The Israel Ophthalmological Society has for these purposes organised the heads of the 17 departments in Israel into a Committee for the Prevention of Blindness. Israel has unique advantages for the investigation of the epidemiological aspects of these diseases. The population is large enough for statistical validities and yet small enough for good organisation on a national scale. About half of its population derives from Europe and the Americas and about half from Oriental countries. The study in depth of these specific causes of blindness in Israel and the Institute's organised survey of all cases of blindness in Israel will inform us of our most pressing eye problems and may suggest the measure advisable to prevent them.

THE INSTITUTE AND APPLIED DEPARTMENT RESEARCH

On one hand the epidemiological studies organized by the Institute will help determine aspects of the most pressing eye problems and perhaps suggest
202

the measures most advisable to prevent them; and, on the other hand, the Institute will try by stimulating interest and by grants, to initiate within eye departments throughout Israel, laboratory and clinical researches dealing with certain of the problems revealed by the epidemiological studies. The stimulation of such applied researches requires means which we do not have at present, except in isolated respects. It is hoped that means will be found to develop these applied researches.

SERVICES FOR PREVENTION OF OCULAR DISEASE

Preventive ophthalmology, like curative ophthalmology, is built on three pillars — knowledge, teaching and service. Service can be defined as the application of existing knowledge by persons who have been taught its importance and use. It is obviously of primary concern to all of us.

There is not yet sufficient knowledge regarding the large majority of the causes of blindness to make possible the organisation of special preventive services for them. These causes include diabetic retinopathy, macular diseases (degenerative and inflammatory), occlusive vascular disease of the retina, detachment of retina, etc. These causes account for about 80% of adult blindness in developed countries and are the subject of research. On the other hand there is accumulated sufficient knowledge regarding glaucoma, certain congenital and inherited diseases to justify possible preventive services in clinics, kindergartens or schools. The role of the Institute is to propose such services where there is sufficient knowledge available, and to advise in their organisation and to assess the results.

LEGISLATION FOR PREVENTION OF OCULAR DISEASES

The Institute will endeavour to initiate legislation for the enforcement of measures important for prevention of eye disease. These will include provision for the prevention of laboratory accidents in school and factory and injuries from children's toys, etc.; the possible need for compulsory vision examination at kindergarten age in order to reveal conditions such as amblyopia; and other measures which are under consideration.

EDUCATION IN PREVENTION FOR THE OPHTHALMOLOGIST, MEDICAL PRACTITIONER AND THE PUBLIC

One of the main functions of the Institute will be to attempt to introduce into the teaching of ophthalmology the concept of prevention as a primary attitude in addition to the usual attitudes of the laboratory and the clinic. This teaching of undergraduates or of specialists in training, has been made difficult because of the lack of easily available sources of information. There is therefore being prepared in the Institute a textbook on prevention in ophthalmology.

It is planned to prepare and to distribute to eye centres in Israel and elsewhere a quarterly bulletin drawing attention to what, in current literature, is new in the prevention of eye diseases. Articles will be prepared for the general medical press. In addition, information will be prepared suitable for the public which can be distributed to the press or form the subject of lectures for lay persons. This information could deal in an easily understood way with subjects as amblyopia, glaucoma, cataract, etc. As it becomes possible, short films dealing with such themes may be made.

BLIND PREVENTION IN DEVELOPING COUNTRIES

The Institute will play its role in the world problems of prevention. Close cooperation will be maintained with the Department of Ophthalmology of the Hebrew University Hadassah Medical School, which under the chairmanship of PROF. ZAUBERMAN is carrying out its unique programme of help to developing countries. During the past 14 years this department has sent over 30 of its staff on ophthalmic missions to Liberia, Tanzania, Ethiopia, Malwai and Rwanda, each mission lasting on an average about two years. Shorter visits have been made to Kenya and Zambia. Over a million patients have been examined and more than 30,000 major operations performed. The Institute's role in this work will be chiefly in teaching and research and its staff will be available to travel to these developing countries where advice on the prevention of blindness is requested.

SUMMARY OF THE PURPOSES OF THE INSTITUTE

The main purposes, of the Jerusalem Institute for the Prevention of Blindness as already indicated in this report may be summarized as follows:
1). To help by research increase knowledge of the main blinding diseases so that they may become the subject of preventive service as well as of research. The Institute is best endowed to help carry out the epidemiological studies, including the therapeutic trials, which are most important parts of the researches.
2). By education, to help increase the number of medical administrators, ophthalmologists, general practitioners and the public who will be aware of this knowledge ad desire its translation into service. This education can best be fulfilled within a medical school.
3). To help advise with preventive services in clinics and in schools.
4). To help where possible preventive services in developing countries. A very large number of the senior members of the 17 eye departments in Israel have had extensive experience of ophthalmology in developing countries.